*A seven-year-old California boy begins suffering from
debilitating exhaustion, double vision, and motor dysfunction.
His personality changes, and he loses his learning skills.
Doctors cannot agree on a diagnosis . . .*

*A Wisconsin plant supervisor admitted to the hospital for
pneumonia suffers massive lung, kidney, and liver deterioration.
Soon he can no longer speak, and is put on life support . . .*

*In Japan, a feverish, convulsive three-month-old is rushed to the
emergency room, where he lapses into a coma . . .*

In *The Virus Within,* award-winning journalist Nicholas Regush
tells the story of HHV-6, a vicious predator that lies dormant
within almost all of us. He shows why it is the key to
understanding AIDS, multiple sclerosis, chronic fatigue
syndrome, and many other serious and fatal illnesses.

He tells us why no one wants to talk about it . . .
and why it is a growing health threat worldwide.

NICHOLAS REGUSH is an award-winning and Emmy-nominated
medical and science journalist at ABC News, where he produces
segments for *World News Tonight with Peter Jennings.* He also
writes the popular "Second Opinion" column on health and medical issues for ABCNEWS.com. A reporter at the *Montreal Gazette*
for twelve years, Regush has written investigative pieces for *Mother
Jones* and *Equinox.* He has appeared on numerous radio and television shows. He lives in New York and Canada.

THE VIRUS WITHIN

A COMING EPIDEMIC

Nicholas Regush

A PLUME BOOK

PLUME
Published by the Penguin Group
Penguin Putnam Inc., 375 Hudson Street, New York, New York 10014, U.S.A.
Penguin Books Ltd, 27 Wrights Lane, London W8 5TZ, England
Penguin Books Australia Ltd, Ringwood, Victoria, Australia
Penguin Books Canada Ltd, 10 Alcorn Avenue, Toronto, Ontario, Canada M4V 3B2
Penguin Books (N.Z.) Ltd, 182-190 Wairau Road, Auckland 10, New Zealand

Penguin Books Ltd, Registered Offices:
Harmondsworth, Middlesex, England

Published by Plume, a member of Penguin Putnam Inc.
Previously published in a Dutton edition.

First Plume Printing, March 2001
10 9 8 7 6 5 4 3 2 1

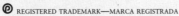 REGISTERED TRADEMARK—MARCA REGISTRADA

The Library of Congress has catalogued the Dutton edition as follows:

Regush, Nicholas M.
The virus within : the coming epidemic / Nicholas Regush.
p. cm.
ISBN 0-525-94534-2 (hc.)
ISBN 0-452-28222-5 (pbk.)
1. Human herpesvirus-6 infections.   I. Title.

QR201.H48 R445 2000
614.5'7—dc21
99–058326

Printed in the United States of America
Original hardcover design by Leonard Telesca

For Barbara, as always and forever

Acknowledgments

First and foremost, I would like to thank my editor, Deb Brody, at Dutton. I was fortunate to have someone to usher in my book who showed such enthusiasm, patience, high-level editing skills, and general all-round smarts in dealing with the likes of me.

And thanks to my agent, Denise Bukowski, for urging me to write this book and even threatening to sit on my doorstep until I completed the manuscript. Denise is a tower of strength, a good friend, and the best agent an author could possibly want. Beware the publisher who doesn't do well by Denise's many authors.

Thanks also to my good friend Alan Morantz from Kingston, Ontario, who reviewed and edited parts of the manuscript and suggested numerous changes. For years I wrote articles for Alan when he was the editor of *Equinox,* Canada's magazine of discovery.

This is an opportunity for me to thank Chuck Ortleb and Neenyah Ostrom, two journalists who spearheaded reporting on HHV-6 for many years for Chuck's now defunct *New York Native.* They both strongly encouraged me to write this book.

As for my colleagues at ABC News who had to put up with me when I needed toothpicks to keep my eyes open, I can only promise them that I'll carry their backpacks up the highest mountain. Well, on second thought . . .

Last, but certainly not least, I want to thank my wife, Barbara, to whom I've dedicated this book. With all due respect to Denise, who would have camped on my doorstep, it was Barbara who gave me the motivation to complete this book in a very short period of time. I couldn't have done it without her daily help, great love, and caring.

Contents

DISCOVERY OF A KILLER

Colorado River Region, California
October 1996

In the fall of 1996, Tina*, in her forties, spiraled ever deeper into depression, suffering from repeated attacks of migraine headaches. Desperate, she offered herself the only prescription that seemed fitting: suicide by drug overdose.

When news of her suicide attempt spread throughout the area, people were shocked. What could drive Tina to such straits? Yet the real tragedy was still on the horizon.

Several months before, Tina had experienced a flurry of flu like symptoms: difficulty in breathing, nausea, diarrhea, fever, and aches all over her body. The symptoms were noted in her medical record, but she made nothing of them. After all, such symptoms are common and transient, usually abating without medical intervention.

In fact, many early symptoms of disease are subtle and do not attract attention until the disease is well established. This is probably why it took so long for Tina's son Len to receive appropriate medical consideration.

---

*Whenever only the first name is used, it is a pseudonym to protect the identity of an individual.

In September 1997, soon after the young boy returned to school after summer vacation, his teacher, Gail, detected a change in his personality from the previous year. Len seemed sad and withdrawn more often than usual, and what had been occasional flashes of anger occurred with increasing frequency. Gail also noticed that his writing skills were in decline. She reasoned that such changes were to be expected in a boy whose mother had attempted suicide.

By early 1998, Len's behavior had deteriorated. In school he was so aggressive with classmates and defiant with his teacher that he was twice suspended. Other times he was so fatigued during afternoon classes that he would fall asleep. On most days he was either too tired or distracted to complete his homework. He was also undergoing physical changes. There were days when he complained of muscle and joint pain and of having weak legs. Once he soiled his clothes and on another occasion could not control his bladder.

Observing Len's erratic and baffling behavior, school officials concluded that he was likely "acting out" in response to a troubled home life. They also decided his schoolwork difficulties were the result of an attention-deficit disorder and that what he needed was old-fashioned school discipline. That approach did not bring any benefit. In April, Len became so aggressive that he threatened his brother, Fred, with a knife. He had also started to have double vision, particularly when he was tired or stressed. Tina, who by this time had awakened to her son's plight, agreed with school officials that Len needed medical testing.

The first warning sign came from a CT (computerized axial tomography) brain scan that revealed some shadowy areas that appeared to be abnormal. Len was then referred by the hospital to a neurologist, who began a more detailed medical investigation. The neurological exam, which included tests for muscle tone and strength, revealed nothing of concern except for swelling in both eyes of his optic disc, the small blind spot on the surface of the retina. The swelling usually occurs when increased pressure is applied from the brain to the optic disc; nerves that surround the optic nerves from the disc are connected to nerve-covering sheaths of the brain.

Hoping for a clearer look at Len's brain, his doctor requested an MRI (magnetic resonance imaging) scan that can produce more detailed images than the CT. The MRI revealed, in the words of the doctor, "fairly extensive white matter disease present with a frontal lobe predominance." Though the "white matter"—the inner areas of the brain rich in nerve fibers—appeared to be diseased, only when sample tissue was removed from Len's frontal lobe a few weeks later did it become evident that the white matter nerve cells had holes and looked like Swiss cheese.

While the tests continued, the only therapy offered was steroids to ease the swelling in the eyes and opiates to tame the headaches he was having. Len's mysterious condition continued to deteriorate rapidly. Soon he could no longer walk without help. He felt wiped out much of the day and had severe headaches. He developed speech impediments and an abnormal sensitivity to light. His teacher, Gail, who visited Len at home, found making emotional contact with him increasingly difficult. Tina feared the worst.

Over the next three months, doctors at several medical centers were asked to consult on the case. Their reviews of biopsy materials led to conflicting opinions. One doctor suggested Len was suffering from a tumor while others thought that some of his nerve fibers were being damaged because they were losing their protective myelin sheaths.

But not one of the doctors initially involved in the case thought of searching for a virus that could be hiding well camouflaged in the pieces of tissue extracted from Len's frontal lobe.

**Milwaukee, Wisconsin
November 1988**

Donald Carrigan sat at his cluttered desk in his cramped office at the Medical College of Wisconsin, reviewing the medical chart of Fred, a 37-year-old man who worked as a supervisor at a water-treatment facility. A colleague, an infectious disease specialist, had asked Carrigan, director of the Diagnostic Virology Laboratory and an expert in detecting viruses, to get involved in the puzzling case. Fred's first symptoms were a fever, sore throat, and cough. Except for being a smoker and having had surgery for an aneurysm, a swollen blood vessel, in the brain, his medical history appeared clean.

Three days after the onset of symptoms, a chest X ray revealed lung abnormalities suggesting pneumonia. He was treated with penicillin to fight off infection, but his health instead deteriorated. Two days later he was admitted to the hospital with additional symptoms, including shivering, a fast rate of breathing, an inadequate flow of oxygen to his tissues, and signs of mental confusion.

Doctors immediately inserted a breathing tube in his windpipe so that proper amounts of oxygen could get to his lungs. They gave him antibiotics known to be effective against a wide range of bacteria and also erythromycin, which is generally used to treat skin, chest, throat, and ear infections, but also Legionnaires' disease, which by then was considered tops on the list of possible causes of his condition.

Legionnaires' is a type of pneumonia that first came to medical attention in 1976 in a Philadelphia hotel, where an outbreak killed 29 members of the American Legion attending a convention. The suspected culprit was a bacterium that scientists at the Centers for Disease Control in Atlanta identified and named Legionella pneumophila, which breeds in water or moist areas such as air-conditioning systems and shower nozzles. Infection is said to be caused by inhaling droplets of water contaminated by the bacterium.

The Milwaukee doctors thought Fred had contracted Legionnaires' disease. Lung, urine, and blood tests indicated strong signs of L. pneumophila.

But even when Rifampin, an antibacterial drug similar to an antibiotic, was added to the treatment regimen, Fred's condition continued to worsen. His kidneys, organs that filter blood and remove waste products from the body, failed, and he required dialysis. His liver began to lose its ability to regulate the main chemicals in his blood. He lost function of his arms and legs. He couldn't urinate. He was placed on life support and could no longer speak.

Further tests showed inflammation and thickening of the tiny air sacs in both lungs, causing them to become less elastic and less efficient. There was also more scarring and thickening of deep-lung tissue, causing shortness of breath.

While all these problems were associated with Legionnaires' disease, Fred wasn't responding to the conventional treatment. Why not? Carrigan asked himself. He lived for opportunities to solve mysteries like this. Science was his life, and nothing was more exciting to him than systematically following a set of clues. In fact, he would much rather spend time in his lab than do just about anything else.

There were no pictures of family or loved ones on Donald Carrigan's office desk. Most scientists, even those in the tiniest of lab stations, want to remind themselves that there is more to life than working until midnight amidst test tubes, microscopes, and flow hoods. To Carrigan, such sentiments simply didn't compute. He was accustomed to being a loner. And good riddance to a marriage that failed and family members that he had stopped seeing many years ago.

So no one among his associates was ever surprised to see him arrive at the lab in the morning, his forty-something lanky frame casually attired, and his silvering ponytail defying convention.

On this particular day, Carrigan focused on the disturbing fact that the patient had almost no lymphocytes, white blood cells critical to the proper functioning of the body's immune system. These cells go on the attack when foreign microbes invade the body.

Tests had already ruled out a wide range of other infections, including influenza A and B and the measles virus. Fred had even been tested for cytomegalovirus, Epstein-Barr virus, and herpes simplex, three common herpes viruses.

Given that the patient's immune system was malfunctioning and his body's lack of response to treatment, Carrigan wondered if he had AIDS. So he conducted the appropriate tests but found no sign of HIV.

What was going on here?

Questions in science are not always answered directly. Sure, lightbulbs do turn on, but medical sleuthing also works in strange ways. Researchers often speak of "serendipity" or an "accident." They are focused on one thing and discover something far different or even more important. Sometimes finding the answer comes from having the patience to study a clue and the self-confidence and creativity to act on a hunch. These were attributes that would carry Donald Carrigan on a trail of clues leading beyond what anyone could have expected.

To say that Donald Carrigan is not the typical science or medical type would be an understatement. Growing up in the sixties, he was pretty wild. Still, a biology teacher at a large high school in the suburbs of Dallas pointed out that a life spent carousing with toughs and drug abusers might turn out to be a tad limited in scope. The teacher let him help out on weekends with research on freshwater mussels, and he discovered that he enjoyed wading through muddy lakes, filling his notebooks with observations. In any event, there was still quality time left over for drugs and sex.

Graduating in 1970, he went on to Cal Tech, where he combined "partying like crazy" with studies in microbiology. As his final year was coming to an end, Carrigan's academic advisers encouraged him to switch his focus from biology to medicine upon graduation. He instead decided he wanted to spend his life in a lab. Most of all he wanted to study viruses and bacteria.

After entering a graduate experimental pathology program at the University of San Diego, though, an unforeseen lack of funds forced students to concentrate mainly on dissecting fish. Carrigan soon dropped out. He ended up with a lab job back at Cal Tech, where he spent most of his time grinding up rabbit spleens for an expensive research project he came to believe bordered on worthless.

One day, as he scanned through a variety of journals at the library, he came across a reference to ongoing research at the University of California at San Francisco. Ken Johnson, a virologist, was exploring the link between the measles virus and neurological damage. Intrigued by the idea, he wrote Johnson a letter asking to serve as a graduate student under his supervision. Johnson was impressed and began making inquiries about Carrigan. Some of the letters of reference weren't particularly flattering. Carrigan was headstrong, said one. Carrigan didn't collaborate well. He basically wasn't a team player. He was very independent. But yes, he was very smart.

Johnson, who was independent-minded himself and not one to suffer baby-sitting a graduate student, took Carrigan in. Soon, exploring biological territory that Johnson had charted, Carrigan identified a new form of measles virus. In 1980 he had a paper, essentially his doctoral dissertation, published by the *Proceedings of the National Academy of Sciences*. It detailed how this new variation of the measles virus caused a chronic inflammation of the spinal cord in hamsters.

Carrigan saw this result as further evidence that a virus could cause disease in the central nervous system. At the time there was a lot of scientific speculation that viruses would prove to be important in progressive nervous system diseases, including multiple sclerosis, in which the protective coverings of nerve fibers (the myelin) in the brain and spinal cord are destroyed. Indeed, Carrigan suggested in the paper that the condition in the hamsters studied bore some resemblance to certain forms of MS. The ultimate death of tissue in both the hamster disease and MS involved cell changes within the tissue and destruction of nerve fiber coverings.

Was measles a trigger for MS? Carrigan thought the idea sufficiently compelling to commit himself to this research path. When Johnson accepted a position at the University of Maryland, Carrigan followed, bringing along his federal government funding on measles virus. By 1987 he had extended his findings on the new measles virus, showing it could damage the brain as well as the spinal cord.

Soon after his new paper was published, his personal life began to fall apart. His marriage went sour, ending in divorce. He became depressed. He grew disenchanted with the measles research. It wasn't progressing quickly enough. Perhaps he was after the wrong virus. He started getting into his old bad habits.

Unexpectedly, he was offered a position at the reputable, if not well-known, Medical College of Wisconsin in Milwaukee, situated in a suburban 248-acre, park-like campus. He could continue his measles research, if he wished, explore new subjects, and head a diagnostic virology lab.

Carrigan wasn't thrilled with the idea of living in Milwaukee, an industrial city of 630,000, considered the beer capital of the nation. Because it is located on the western shore of Lake Michigan, where the Milwaukee, Menomonee, and Kinnickinnic rivers meet, it is often foggy and very cold, not to mention the heavy snowfall. But he accepted the offer, buoyed by feelings of starting fresh.

He promptly began new viral research, this time focusing on the possibility that a virus could trigger schizophrenia, generally thought to be a group of illnesses involving disturbances in emotions, thinking, and behavior. He would continue his measles research as well, which was when he received the call from his colleague in infectious diseases, asking him to do some tests on Fred.

*   *   *

Carrigan might have shrugged off the negative HIV tests he ran on Fred. He might have closed the book on the case. Instead he studied his HIV cultures—the nutrient materials used to grow and reproduce microbes—again and again. No, there certainly wasn't any HIV, but what he finally discovered fascinated him.

Carrigan saw strange, balloon-like cells coming up in the culture. He had no idea what they were.

He remembered vaguely that during one of his library visits, he had seen pictures of peculiar cells in a paper published in an edition of *Science*. In 1986, researchers from Robert Gallo's laboratory at the National Cancer Institute had identified a new virus, taken from an AIDS patient. Carrigan looked up the journal and there they were, the same big, peculiar cells. They appeared to be identical to those in his culture. The new virus had apparently caused cells to balloon.

Then what about Fred, who was presumed to have Legionnaires' disease? Was it this newly identified virus that was wreaking havoc with his immune system?

As Fred drifted perilously close to death, the disease suddenly took a turn for the better. Shortly after he was given high doses of corticosteroid drugs, his breathing improved significantly, and within a week he was taken off life-support systems. Days later, dialysis was discontinued, and he began speaking to hospital staff. Before long, he was well enough to be transferred to a rehabilitation hospital.

Donald Carrigan was perplexed. Why had steroids—powerful anti-inflammatory drugs—been so effective? Did they target an infection other than the L. pneumophila associated with Legionnaires' disease? And what of the odd, balloon-shaped cells he had observed: were they missing pieces of the puzzle? Determined to find the answer, Carrigan contacted the scientists at the National Cancer Institute who had discovered the peculiar cells and asked for help. He needed their test materials to determine if the cells he had seen in his culture medium had been damaged by the same virus.

*   *   *

Those "juicy" cells, as the NCI scientists called them, were keys to an important discovery that came to light soon after the scientific world had largely settled on the theory that a virus which became known as HIV (Human Immunodeficiency Virus) was the cause of AIDS. One of the scientists at NCI working closely with Robert Gallo, whose lab had contributed to the discovery of HIV, was Bangladesh-born Syed Zaki Salahuddin. In the aftermath of that discovery, Salahuddin began to spend more of his lab time investigating AIDS-related lymphomas. Lymphomas are cancers of the immune system; they overwhelm small filtering organs called lymph nodes. AIDS patients are particularly vulnerable to a form that invades B-cells. These are cells that produce antibodies that circulate in the blood and target foreign substances. When lymphoma strikes, a type of malignant B-cell grows rapidly until it crowds out others, thus hindering the patient's overall ability to fight infection with antibodies. For AIDS sufferers, such a cancer diminishes their already overwhelmed defenses. It had long been suspected that the trigger for lymphoma was the Epstein-Barr virus, a commonly occurring member of the herpes family. Salahuddin, however, had a hunch that the culprit might be an unusual form of Epstein-Barr.

Working away in the lab, Salahuddin and NCI colleague Dharam Ablashi demonstrated that people with AIDS usually had high amounts of antibodies against Epstein-Barr present in blood serum, suggesting that their immune systems had mounted an attack against the infection. There were also higher than usual signs of the virus circulating in their plasma, the liquid part of the blood. But such encouraging signs that their research was on the right track were short-lived. They soon discovered that AIDS patients with lymphoma were indistinguishable from control subjects without AIDS and malignancy. Perhaps Epstein-Barr was not the cause after all.

Their experiments then took an unexpected turn. During the standard laboratory procedures that are followed to detect viruses, Salahuddin and Ablashi had induced the division of white blood cells called leukocytes from the blood of AIDS patients. Some of the cells ballooned, although it took an experienced eye to detect the phenomenon. One of their colleagues referred to such large and oddly shaped cells—clearly different from those typically said to be infected only with HIV—as "juicy," and the label stuck.

The NCI scientists considered it likely that juicy cells were the result of infection by an unknown virus. Further tests confirmed that they could, for example, transmit the infection to white blood cells taken from human umbilical cord blood, which is free of the types of infections that can be found in adult blood samples. They were thus able to reproduce the juicy cells.

Closer study suggested at first that juicy cells were immature B-cells. Since the new virus appeared to have a propensity to attack this type of cell, NCI researchers named it HBLV, for Human B-Cell Lymphotropic Virus. In a paper published in the journal *Science* in October 1986, they detailed how the virus was isolated and included pictures of the juicy cells. In a second paper in the same edition, they presented biological, including genetic, evidence that HBLV was likely a new herpes virus.

In August 1987, the papers were followed by impressive data, this time in the British journal *The Lancet,* showing that HBLV appeared to be capable of causing more damage than previously documented. Research headed by Robert Downing at the PHLS Center of Applied Microbiological Research in Porton Down, England, revealed that the newly identified virus was also targeting other types of cells, including T-4 lymphocytes (also referred to as CD4s), key cells of the immune system. Researchers who had isolated the virus from white blood cell cultures of Ugandans with AIDS, using molecular probes for HBLV developed at NCI, suggested it would be appropriate to rename the virus LHV, for Lymphotropic Human Herpesvirus. A month later, NCI researchers reported in *The Lancet* that they too had discovered that HBLV had a special attraction for T-4 cells. They proposed their own new name for the virus: Human Herpes Virus-6 or HHV-6 (the sixth herpes virus that had been isolated).

When NCI laboratory research revealed the extent of HHV-6's destructive power, Robert Gallo began to speak out about the implications. On May 10, 1988, at the annual meeting of the American Society for Microbiology in Miami, he told an audience that HHV-6 had been found along with HIV in T-4 cells, and speculated that the new herpes virus could be a "co-factor" in AIDS. One month later, at an international AIDS conference in Stockholm, he explained that HHV-6 killed T-4 cells in the test tube more effectively than did HIV, and said the new herpes virus could cause massive cell death. Gallo reasoned that HHV-6 infection might help speed up the HIV-led breakdown of the immune system in AIDS, although he cautioned that the NCI research on HHV-6 was still preliminary.

After the early papers on the new herpes virus were published, numerous researchers contacted Gallo, Salahuddin, and Ablashi to report that they too were encountering juicy cells, not only in their cultures from AIDS patients but from sufferers of immune system–related illnesses, from young children with seizures, blood disorders, and kidney problems; from individuals who had received organ transplants; and from people diagnosed with a mysterious malady known as chronic fatigue syndrome. Some of the researchers reported that they had seen juicy cells in cultures taken even from apparently healthy individuals. The question then became whether or not the juicy cells that had been observed in such a wide range of cultures were infected with HHV-6.

Donald Carrigan was one of many scientists who received the NCI test materials that could help detect the newly identified virus. Painstaking laboratory work soon convinced him that the virus was involved in Fred's case. Carrigan found it in a blood sample that had been drawn during the acute phase of Fred's illness, when his symptoms abruptly became intense. A biopsy of Fred's lung tissue showed lymphocytes and other cells were infected throughout by HHV-6. Studies of the virus with an electron microscope and antibody tests further confirmed its presence. And so it was highly likely that the herpes virus had somehow contributed to the pneumonia.

In reaching their conclusion, Carrigan and his colleagues had also taken into account that steroid treatment had rapidly cleared the pneumonia; they had shown in lab tests that steroids had the ability to stop HHV-6 from reproducing. They suspected that the virus, in attacking lymphocytes and other immune cells that fight inflammation, may have contributed to the virulence of the pneumonia. The steroids, besides possibly having attacked the HHV-6, had also fought off the inflammation in the lungs.

What exact role HHV-6 played in Fred's illness remained a mystery. Carrigan was determined to learn everything he could about the virus. It not only appeared to have the ability to infect the same cells that HIV did, but also to infect the lungs of an adult who developed pneumonia. What else could HHV-6 do?

By taking this road, he would find himself at the heart of a major scientific adventure with all that this entails—the spirit of extraordinary discovery as well as the hardship of controversy.

Few were as ready for such a journey as Donald Carrigan.

AN HIV CHAMPION
AND HIS DETRACTORS

About 700 miles from Donald Carrigan's cramped office in Milwaukee, a taxi dropped me off at the National Cancer Institute, situated in a huge campus among the scores of other science and medical buildings that make up the National Institutes of Health. I had come to visit Robert Gallo, whose lab had helped discover HIV. He was also the leader of the team that had discovered HHV-6. I wanted to question him about both viruses.

I had met Gallo two years earlier to discuss some concerns by scientists that both he and Luc Montagnier (and Jay Levy too) had perhaps reached the conclusion too quickly that HIV was in fact the cause of AIDS. On that occasion Gallo had revealed some bitterness about those assertions but had remained calm in his attempts to convince me that the virus was indeed the culprit.

On this frosty fall day, Gallo revealed why he had earned the reputation of sometimes being hostile, arrogant, and uncompromising. "Look, HIV causes AIDS, end of story, and anyone who thinks otherwise belongs on another planet," Gallo barked menacingly. Small and wiry, with graying hair, Gallo, age 52, gestured wildly and looked daggers at me. It was peculiar behavior for a sci-

entist who probably thought of himself as a prime candidate for
the Nobel Prize.

Unlike Carrigan, who worked in relative obscurity, Gallo had
movie star recognition in the scientific community. His picture
hung among the gliterati in a chichi Mexican restaurant in
Bethesda, a short hike from his lab. Unlike Carrigan, who had to
beg, borrow, and steal for research assistance from Medical College, Gallo had everything his heart could desire: well-equipped
laboratories; a steady flow of money for experimentation; post-
doctoral students to investigate his research requests; a team of
collaborators; and a legion of science reporters eager to present his
views on HIV and AIDS. Yet if Gallo had all this, why was he so
worked up on this day? I had brought up the name of his sharpest
critic: Peter Duesberg.

A microbiologist at the University of California at Berkeley,
Duesberg was relentlessly attacking Gallo's view of HIV as a killer.
The point I had raised in particular was Duesberg's questioning of
Gallo's recent interest in so-called co-factors that helped HIV overwhelm the immune system. Anyone who bothered searching for a
co-factor, Duesberg reasoned, was obviously unclear of the actual
cause of a disease. He lectured to colleagues at scientific conferences
on what he termed the "AIDS boondoggle," and pointed out that
the consequences were dire. Billions of scientific research and health
care dollars would be wasted. Attacking HIV to treat AIDS would
be ineffective and lead to many thousands of needless deaths. The
test for exposure to HIV—used to screen blood donations or flag
people at risk for AIDS—would result in discrimination, with some
losing their jobs and others even committing suicide out of fear. In
the end, when the HIV hoax came to be exposed, Duesberg said, science would suffer an unprecedented loss of trust.

Gallo's response was unequivocal: "I can't respond without
shrieking." He added in a calmer voice, "You know, Peter is only
seeking publicity. Peter is very smart, but he really doesn't know
what he's talking about when he speaks about AIDS."

There is one thing that can be said with confidence about
Robert Gallo: he's no quitter. Once convinced that trailblazing a

particular scientific path will reap rewards, Gallo soldiers on. He has made a career of backing the wild card, dismissing stinging personal failure as an inevitable feature of modern science. In the process, he has made it known to his detractors that he does not back away from a fight.

Gallo's commitment to medicine began at the age of 12, when his sister Judy died of leukemia. Her painful, progressive demise left him feeling helpless and devastated. Medical research would eventually become his way of better understanding the beast that had killed her.

Gallo joined the National Cancer Institute in 1965, at the age of 29. He followed a well-marked route: majoring in biology at Providence College, graduating from the Thomas Jefferson University School of Medicine in Philadelphia, and completing a one-year research fellowship at the University of Chicago. At NCI, after serving the required year as a doctor, mainly in a pediatric leukemia unit, he turned his attention to research, which included the study of white blood-cell growth in the leukemias.

Before long Gallo's attention focused on a bold new thrust in cancer research, studying a family of viruses that possibly infected humans and caused cancer. The idea had first developed in 1909, when studies showed that tumors could be induced in otherwise healthy chickens by injecting them with tumor tissue from chickens that had developed cancers of soft tissue. Such an invader, which grew and reproduced only inside a living cell, was called an RNA tumor virus. That is because its genetic code, as is the case with some viruses, was made up of RNA (ribonucleic acid), in contrast to a virus that has DNA (deoxyribonucleic acid, the genetic material of most living organisms). But when similar experiments failed in other animals, the idea lost favor. It resurfaced only in the 1950s with a stream of new animal experiments, usually conducted by veterinarians.

Then in 1970, scientists discovered an enzyme, a biological catalyst, in cancer cells that helped researchers find fingerprints of these RNA tumor viruses. The enzyme, which became known as reverse transcriptase, enabled an RNA-based virus to convert itself to the DNA of its host cell's DNA nucleus—thus the "transcription." (Previously, conventional thinking held that DNA could convert to RNA but not the other way.) It was then assumed that the detection of the enzyme could serve as a marker for an RNA virus. In other words, detecting the presence of the enzyme would suggest that an RNA tumor virus—or retrovirus, as it came to be known—had made an appearance.

The discovery was good timing for cancer researchers. In 1971 President Richard Nixon launched his war on cancer by initiating the National Cancer Act, which authorized funds for a small army of scientists. Retroviruses took their place in the research pantheon with other potential culprits of the disease. Gallo, promoted to head a new department that would devote itself to the hunt, chose the leukemias as his focus. He was determined to find a retrovirus infecting leukemic cells. It was the opportunity of a lifetime.

In 1972 he and colleagues published evidence of reverse transcriptase in human leukemia, but few scientists were impressed. A quick study, Gallo realized that he would make an impact only by actually isolating a retrovirus and somehow growing it in the laboratory.

In 1975 he announced the first isolation of a human retrovirus, named HL-23, from a leukemia patient. Unfortunately for Gallo, the isolate was not what it seemed to be. He sent samples to scientists for their review, and the bad news was presented at a scientific meeting in Hershey, Pennsylvania. There was no HL-23, only three animal viruses, from a monkey, gibbon, and baboon. HL-23 was a laboratory contaminant.

Gallo was so shocked by the turn of events that he even considered the possibility that his work had been sabotaged. In any case, he was a laughingstock. Some cancer researchers even called his work a hunt for "human rumor viruses."

One reason for the doubts about the supposed link between retroviruses and human cancers stemmed from the growing understanding that humans have a sizable amount of genetic sequences of such viruses entwined with their own genetic code, possibly resulting from infections originating in ancient times.

Carrying retroviruses, therefore, is part of what it means to be human. There was certainly no evidence that such sequences were triggering cancer in humans.

While considering so-called "endogenous" retroviruses to be harmless, Gallo insisted that "exogenous," or external, retroviruses were capable of inserting some of their genes into cells and triggering abnormal behavior, namely tumor development. In fact, one reason why scientists such as Gallo even entertained the possibility that retroviruses could cause cancer was that they did not appear to kill cells but merely altered their functioning.

Gallo continued his search, and in 1980 he turned up what he presented as the first human T-cell leukemia virus (HTLV). This was a retrovirus first taken from the cells of several leukemia patients and then grown in the lab. Despite the fact that other leukemic cells produced no HTLV, Gallo was now focused on finding a disease for the virus. Along with some collaborators, he managed to locate it on an island in Japan, in parts of Africa, and in the Caribbean. Tests showed that there appeared to be a niche for HTLV in these regions, and there was also a particular type of leukemia. Gallo proposed that one was related to the other: HTLV caused the disease. He continued to take this stand even as evidence filtered in that signs of the virus could be detected in perfectly healthy people. In response, Gallo argued that it would take many years for the leukemia to develop. According to some of Gallo's critics, there is still no convincing evidence for this theory.

HTLV (later renamed HTLV-1) was the very same virus Gallo first considered in 1982 as possibly causing AIDS. He and Myron Essex, a virologist at Harvard University, had considered the idea that people with AIDS seemed to be suffering symptoms similar to those of immune-suppressed cats that were infected with a leukemia retrovirus. Gallo figured that because the T-4 cells of the immune system were targets in AIDS, an HTLV virus might qualify as a candidate because of its attraction to the same immune cells. He and Essex then pursued the theory that HTLV-1 was the likely cause of AIDS.

In the end, though, all Gallo could muster was the meager finding that HTLV-1 genes could be detected in the DNA of T-4 cells
in two of 33 AIDS patients and that the virus had been isolated
from the cells of another patient. All Essex could add was the finding that antibodies to HTLV-1 could be found in about 25 percent
of people with AIDS and enlarged lymph nodes. (Not published
until 1984, due to lack of interest, was a small but arresting study
conducted by scientists from New York, Nebraska, and Japan,
showing in separate laboratory tests that there was no sign of
HTLV-1 in the blood of 15 people with AIDS and at risk for AIDS
in New York City.)

Meanwhile, in May 1983, Luc Montagnier and his associates at
the Paris-based Pasteur Institute reported the detection of an unknown virus in the swollen lymph nodes of a patient considered
at risk for contracting AIDS. They named the virus LAV, for
lymphadenopathy-associated virus. Montagnier did not actually
claim to have proven that his virus caused AIDS, so to encourage
further study he sent samples of the tissue cultures to Gallo at NCI.

Gallo himself switched gears, forsaking HTLV-1 in favor of
HTLV-3, a virus that the U.S. government announced on April 23,
1984 (with Gallo standing proudly at the press conference), as the
likely cause of AIDS. This event occurred the day after *The New
York Times* published a report in which scientists at the Centers
for Disease Control in Atlanta suggested that the Pasteur scientists
were closing in on the cause of AIDS. As it happened, HTLV-3,
which Gallo and his team claimed to have found independently,
turned out to be almost identical to the French virus sent to Gallo
for examination purposes.

Both scientific teams said their viruses targeted T-4 lymphocytes, a subgroup of white blood cells that are key components of
the body's defense against foreign microbial invasion. Given such
similarities and the high stakes in AIDS research, Gallo's announcement touched off a firestorm in the science community. In 1985 the
Pasteur Institute said Gallo had approximated its virus, and it took
two years of often tense negotiation before a compromise settlement
was reached. Both Montagnier and Gallo were granted the title of

"co-discoverer" of the virus that became classified as HIV. Ulti-mately, the French retrovirus would be seen as the sole "AIDS virus."

The entire idea quickly attracted critics, in particular Peter Duesberg. In 1985, at a science conference in West Germany, Gallo introduced Peter Duesberg as a man of extraordinary en-ergy, unusual honesty, an enormous sense of humor, and a rare critical sense "that often makes us look twice, then a third time, at a conclusion many of us believed to be foregone."

The Californian—like Gallo, small and feisty—was given to wearing canary yellow dress shirts or rock magazine T-shirts at sci-entific meetings. Soon he was attacking "Big Bob," the "head of the AIDS mafia," as Duesberg often referred to Gallo, and refer-ring to the "Big Mistake," namely the Gallo-supported misdirec-tion of AIDS research.

In 1986 Duesberg was invited by the Fogarty International Center of the National Institutes of Health to spend a year doing whatever research struck his fancy. Duesberg was already a much honored recipient of numerous high-profile research prizes and a newly elected member of the science hall of fame, better known as the National Academy of Sciences.

Duesberg also had the reputation of being a maverick, who was even willing to turn on his own discoveries. Gallo and other can-cer virus researchers were far from pleased when Duesberg, who had helped to spearhead the hunt for retroviruses in the 1970s, de-cided the effort didn't add up to much. These retroviruses, which he had proposed—and even demonstrated under laboratory con-ditions—could insert certain genes into cells to cause cancer, were actually harmless in humans, he had later concluded, and were content to live harmoniously integrated in human cells. Could they cause cancer? There was no evidence for this whatsoever.

Duesberg, believing Gallo and the other cancer virus hunters were now repeating their failures in AIDS research, decided to spend his Fogarty year in the library at NIH, examining the evi-dence in support of a retroviral cause. He didn't find it compelling in the least, and wrote up his conclusions in a lengthy review article in the journal *Cancer Research*. Initially, there was no response, but as word slowly spread throughout academe, the invectives came flying, particularly from Gallo.

Duesberg asked some very basic questions that had to be addressed. Above all, he questioned the proposition that the cause of AIDS is a retrovirus that kills T-cells. He had searched the available scientific data and found no evidence that the virus was active in cells, even in people who were dying of AIDS. How could this be if the virus was a killer? It seemed that the virus was just sitting there, doing nothing, which is exactly what he expected a retrovirus to be doing. Furthermore, Duesberg was outraged that AIDS scientists had embraced as a causal agent a virus that infected so few cells. After all, AIDS was supposed to occur when T-4 cells were wiped out of the body's immune system.

Duesberg was also surprised to discover that AIDS scientists were placing a high premium on testing positive for HIV. Traditionally such a sign that the body's immune system has developed a reaction (antibodies) to a virus is seen as evidence that the threat of infection is over. It is akin to vaccination. But AIDS scientists, for reasons that Duesberg could not fathom, viewed a positive test as a sign that AIDS was likely to develop in the future.

Underlying Duesberg's discontent with AIDS science was their insistence that the "AIDS virus," after causing a quickly passing flu-like illness, became "latent" (inactive) possibly for many years before it stirred to create havoc in the body. This was why in some individuals the disease was taking years before it graduated from a positive antibody status to AIDS. But, asked Duesberg, where was the proof for such a theory? He characterized this belief in a "slow" virus in humans as a sign of "slow virologists at work."

This "slow human virus" concept had its origins in 1957 in the exotic climes of New Guinea, when an NIH scientist, Carleton Gajdusek, uncovered a disease called "kuru," which attacked the brain to paralyze and then kill its victims. Gajdusek thought the disease was infectious and had strong suspicions that it was transmitted via acts of cannibalism, when the natives ate the brains of relatives. But no virus could be detected, or any typical signs that a virus had invaded the body, including such biological markers as inflammation and immune reaction. There was still no evidence of the virus when Gajdusek returned to NIH and injected mashed-up brains from kuru victims into monkeys by means of holes he drilled through their skulls. But some of the animals eventually did show signs of neurologic disability. A slow virus, Gajdusek claimed, therefore must have done the job and was possibly triggering other devastating neurological diseases, perhaps even including multiple sclerosis and Alzheimer's. Gajdusek was rewarded for his studies on kuru with the Nobel Prize for Medicine in 1976. Duesberg, at a cranky moment, would refer to 1976 as a "slow year for science."

And, of course, Duesberg firmly believed that 1984, the year the cause of AIDS was announced, was also a year that science one day would prefer to forget.

In sum, Duesberg came to conclude that the available data suggested rather that the "AIDS virus" was merely a harmless "passenger" virus, which was part of the body's viral baggage.

By the fall of 1988, Robert Gallo was listening more attentively to Duesberg that HIV might not be killing T-4 cells directly. But he had already considered possible ways HIV could destroy the immune system indirectly. For instance, the immune system in targeting HIV could also create conditions that led to the massacre of T-4 cells. Also, AIDS scientists were pursuing numerous new leads to determine exactly how the T-4 cells were killed. Maybe other viruses, such as HHV-6, played a role in orchestrating the death of these cells.

"Peter typically just doesn't understand that HIV can kill T-4 cells indirectly," Gallo said. "He is not equipped to deal with this kind of thinking."

So why doesn't he meet Duesberg face to face in a public debate?

"I have no time to waste on such things," Gallo replied.

Gallo was not merely being testy when he said he would not debate Duesberg on HIV. His attitude may have helped to quash a debate at the White House that was set for January 19, 1988. Jim Warner, one of President Ronald Reagan's domestic policy advisers, had called the meeting to "deal with some of the doubts in the minds of policy makers," specifically to sort out claims that the scientific establishment had made a major error in concluding that HIV was the cause of AIDS. Warner was concerned that funds spent on AIDS research were being misdirected and hoped the meeting could be the first step to opening new avenues of research. "Those guys at the NIH, including Gallo," he said, "are doing everything possible to avoid addressing challenges to the HIV theory."

Duesberg was invited to the White House meeting. He viewed the debate as an opportunity to publicly deconstruct some of the HIV theory that he believed was on shaky ground. He also wanted to alert policy makers to the need for research on specific risk behaviors among groups that appeared vulnerable to AIDS, particularly gay and bisexual men and intravenous drug users. At the time he believed AIDS was first and foremost a condition that developed when an individual exposed to high amounts of stress and strain suffered a weakened immune system. Duesberg planned to call for research that would focus on "toxic hits" people received that would lead to AIDS. As far as he was concerned, HIV was merely a biological marker, or red flag, that revealed immune damage had occurred. This was why signs of viral infection correlated so well with immune damage—not because the virus caused it but because some other entity temporarily triggered a harmless retroviral reaction, just enough to have its host declared "antibody positive."

Duesberg's concerns about "toxic hits" to cells were not new to discussions on AIDS. Joseph Sonnabend, a New York doctor who was among the first to care for people with AIDS, noticed that gay and bisexual men who engaged in promiscuous and anonymous sex in certain environments—such as bathhouses—were contracting multiple infections. It was unlikely anyone living this way could avoid disease.

By late 1979 many gay men were turning up with low white-cell counts, suggesting possible immune system problems. Their blood proteins were elevated, a sign of chronic infection. Some had swollen lymph nodes, possibly linked to unresolved syphilis or hepatitis B infections. A few had enlarged spleens, another sign of chronic infection. Sonnabend also noted that the majority of the men were passive partners in anal sex, essentially becoming receptacles for infections. His research showed that the degree of immune system suppression they experienced appeared to be related to the number of sexual contacts with different partners. The medical literature of the time also indicated that many gay men used a variety of street drugs such as "poppers" and cocaine that could further weaken the immune system. When AIDS was first identified in 1981, Sonnabend assumed the immune system breakdowns resulted from such a perilous lifestyle.

With gay men as his focus, Sonnabend theorized that at least two stages could lead to the deadly syndrome. The first stage, reversible through lifestyle changes, stemmed from an accumulation of infectious assaults on the body. At some undetermined point, however, the complex biological processes that are unleashed become self-sustaining. The second and irreversible stage ended in a complete breakdown of the immune system, or AIDS.

Sonnabend's core idea that a buildup of immunological problems paves the way for AIDS also led him to reassure society early in the epidemic that generally healthy people are not likely to develop AIDS. In this vein, he wrote that health authorities were defining groups at risk for AIDS much too broadly. For example, he argued that gay men were not equally at risk because only some were involved in the type of sexual promiscuity that led to chronic infections that suppressed body defenses against illnesses.

Sonnabend also pointed to several studies published in 1983 that suggested a blood-clotting agent required by hemophiliacs could suppress the immune system. This is how hemophiliacs were likely developing AIDS, and not via HIV. The product, known as Factor Eight, was being pooled from up to 25,000 blood donors and was mostly made up of foreign proteins that are not essential to blood clotting. Some research suggested that the more foreign proteins a hemophiliac takes into his system, the more likely the immune system becomes suppressed.

Had the debate at the White House occurred, Sonnabend would have asked for research funding to gain a broader understanding of the environments of AIDS sufferers and to better determine what, if any, significant changes had occurred in such environments. Focusing solely on HIV, he believed, would be disastrous medical policy.

A worried Sonnabend had summed up his views in the following manner to me early in the AIDS epidemic: "Medical teachings nowadays have become too hung up on a model of illness that looks for single microbes that cause disease. The bench scientists in their high-tech labs search the body for viruses and then try to find diseases for them. It is the ultimate form of reductionism."

He went further: "Scientists today favor a single-agent theory rather than a broader view of disease because it allows them to work in their labs and work out all the properties of the agent, which is very exciting. But it is not so exciting if it is out of context of more general appreciation of cell biology and biology in general. This approach also moves science away from a study of environmental conditions and lifestyles, in other words, away from the complexities of the world."

Other scientists shared Sonnabend's misgivings about how the use of powerful new tools in molecular biology could result in confusing experimental artifacts with the real world. One scientist, Eleni Papadopulos-Eleopulos from the Royal Perth Hospital in western Australia, offered a strong case for how she believed such confusion had occurred. Like both Sonnabend and Duesberg, she had detected a link among the various groups deemed at risk for AIDS. All groups seemed to have been subjected to major stressors, which Papadopulos-Eleopulos theorized could harm cells sufficiently to lower the body's production of T-4 cells. In the process, she said, damaged cells could give rise to the genetic expression of retroviral sequences already entwined in the cells. And that was what testing was actually measuring, not some so-called infectious HIV that had been spread by blood. Of all the challengers to the HIV theory, Papadopulous-Eleopulos was perhaps the most daring, questioning the very existence of HIV.

Given such attacks, it was not surprising that Gallo perked up when I mentioned HHV-6. Because the herpes virus and HIV infect the same cell and work together, he explained, HHV-6 could be part of a vicious cycle in the body. He was referring to preliminary evidence, notwithstanding HHV-6's striking ability to kill T-4 cells in the laboratory.

Despite his enthusiasm to talk about his role in the detection of HHV-6, though, Gallo was beginning to have mild doubts about the importance of the virus. Data were streaming in from labs around the world, suggesting that HHV-6 might not be so special after all. In fact, it appeared to be a very common infection. And if it was so common, how could it possibly be a player in AIDS?

With hindsight, it is easy to conclude that such reasoning was incomplete. Others would take up the task of investigating HHV-6, and they would be surprised at just how much a common virus could accomplish.

NEW AND EVOLVING CHAMELEONS

Picture a mother tucking in her three-month-old son before a nap. Filled with maternal love, she kisses sweet Yoshizo. Yet within her moist kiss lies a potential viral stowaway that can infiltrate Yoshizo's young body. Wrapped in a shell of proteins and membranes, this type of invader cannot see, smell, hear, or taste. But it does have one invaluable asset: a predator's cunning.

True to its kind, the virus that infected Yoshizo set out to detect telltale chemicals on the surface of target cells in the young boy's body. It then attaches itself to one of these sites. It breaches the cell's protective plasma membrane, advances to the cell's interior and, like a quick-change burglar, sheds its outer coating. Now established in the cell, it begins to churn out its genetic code, its deoxyribonucleic acid (DNA). Tricked into being an accomplice, the cell's machinery makes perfect copies of the foreign virus.

The invader keeps the child's cell alive until it can no longer manufacture new virus. At that point the cell bursts and releases the viral progeny, which infects and begins taking over other cells to make more viruses.

At first the virus's intent is to establish a secure beachhead where it can develop an accommodation with its new host and continue to evolve without incident. It has to fight off early attacks from Yoshizo's immune system. His arsenal of biochemical defenses is deployed to limit the replication of the virus and to flush out the enemy. But this tiny infant will lose the battle.

Before long, outward signs will reveal the turmoil within. On July 28, Yoshizo will develop a fever, accompanied by vomiting and jaundice. One day he seems like a healthy baby and then suddenly, without warning, he appears to be severely ill. And this isn't some peculiar childhood flare-up that will quickly be resolved. Yoshizo will be rushed to a hospital where he will arrive convulsing and in a deep coma apparently related to a destroyed liver. Therapy, including transfusions, will have no beneficial effect. The coma will deepen. Yoshizo will die on August 4.

Koichi Yamanishi, a physician at Osaka University's Research Institute for Microbial Diseases, became involved in Yoshizo's case when it was suspected that the infant's illness resulted from infection by a virus named HHV-6.

A year earlier, Yamanishi and his colleagues at various Japanese health and research facilities had been the first to demonstrate that HHV-6 causes a common childhood disease known by various names, mainly roseola but also exanthem subitum, pseudorubella, and three-day fever. Striking those under the age of four, the illness is marked by a rash on the face, trunk, and even arms and legs of the victim, accompanied by a high fever lasting three to five days. Other common symptoms include drowsiness, irritability, nasal congestion, diarrhea, cough, wheezing, and vomiting.

Less common and more troublesome are seizures, mostly mild but sometimes severe. Though Yoshizo did not develop the characteristic roseola rash, he did acquire the fever, vomiting, drowsiness, and convulsions, enough markers to alert Yamanishi and his colleagues that HHV-6 might be the culprit.

Extensive laboratory tests confirmed their suspicions: HHV-6 appeared responsible for the liver disease, which also likely caused the brain to shut down. The virus's invasion of Yoshizo's brain might have contributed to the coma. The findings were novel and alarming. Previously published reports of HHV-6's role in roseola had been limited mostly to the occurrence of rather mild and transient symptoms.

Never underestimate the influence of a name. Conjuring images of soft flower petals, the term roseola hardly captures the true nature of the disease. Roseola was first officially described in 1910, but another 40 years would pass before researchers seriously investigated it as an infection. Studies in 1950 and 1951 showed that the blood of infants with roseola could be injected into other infants to cause the condition. Because roseola could be spread by blood, scientists of the time believed a virus could be involved, but they were unable to prove their case. They lacked the modern molecular tools to identify viruses, which have become available only in the past two decades.

Only after research into AIDS in the 1980s and the Gallo laboratory's subsequent discovery of HHV-6 would serious attention focus on roseola. Interest in the newly discovered virus led Yamanishi and other scientists to link HHV-6 in blood cells of four infants with roseola. The scientists also detected antibodies to the virus in 10 other infants with the disease, indicating that proteins produced by the body's immune system were reacting to the invader. But most of the research at the time found the virus in combination with only modest illnesses.

There were other reasons why the true measure of HHV-6 was not taken. First, further studies from around the world showed that most individuals who had their blood tested for HHV-6 were turning up antibody positive to the virus, meaning their immune systems at one time had neutralized the infection. After HHV-6 first infects a human host, the antibodies that are made by the body's immune system early in infection persist. They are maintained at lower but detectable levels in more than 90 percent of the adult population. Usually past the age of 40, the levels begin to fall off gradually.

HHV-6's low profile could also be traced to diminishing concern among scientists overall about the role of microbes in human

health. For at least two decades before the virus was detected in
human blood cells, many infectious-disease specialists had been
insisting that humankind had gained the upper hand in its battles
with the microbial world and had largely forced the enemy into retreat. After all, public health advances had ushered in a new era of
clean water and food supplies and better living conditions as well
as antibiotics and vaccines. Smallpox, an infection that had killed
300 million people in the twentieth century alone, had been eradi-
cated, and massively destructive diseases such as bubonic plague,
malaria, tuberculosis, cholera, diphtheria, typhoid, syphilis, and
polio had been beaten back to varying degrees.

Some infectious-disease specialists were even declaring an end
to the global war. Public health officials in the United States,
Canada, and Britain, for instance, announced in the 1970s and
early 1980s that in the developed nations chronic diseases related
to lifestyle had become the new medical battlefield. Smoking,
drinking, poor diet, and automobile accidents were the new ad-
versaries. To many public health officials, the appearance of AIDS
was the exception to the forecasted trend.

Had scientists studying HHV-6 in the summer of 1989 been capable of seeing a few years into the future, they likely would have
been stunned by the evidence revealing the common virus was a
nasty pathogen in children whose immune systems, for one reason
or another, could not protect them against it.

Yoshizo's tragedy was the first report of many that highlighted
an out-of-control infection. Scientists began documenting numerous examples of HHV-6–infected children with roseola developing
moderate to severe illnesses after the initial symptoms, ranging
from blood disorders to heart, lung, liver, and nervous system
damage. Some children would die of HHV-6 infection, often very
swiftly.

Consider the case of 13-month-old Vietnamese-born Nan, a
twin, who by all appearances was healthy and vital before she became ill. The child first developed a fever accompanied by an ear
infection. Offered food, she pushed away her plate. When she was
examined at the emergency room of a local community hospital in
New York state, doctors judged her to be mildly dehydrated and

admitted her for intravenous feeding and antibiotic therapy. Soon after initial treatment, a rash erupted on her face and trunk, and worried doctors stopped her medication. Nan remained feverish.

Because of growing concern, the wasting young patient was transferred to New York University Medical Center in Manhattan. Upon admission, her temperature rose to 105 degrees, her heart pumped at a rapid 130 beats per minute, and the rash on her body expanded beyond her face and trunk to parts of her arms and legs. Ominously, blood crusted on her lips, evidence that her blood vessels were leaking. Immediate treatment at the hospital included drugs to fight infection and boost her immune system. She also received blood transfusions to control hemorrhaging. But intervention was futile: the cellular machinery so critical to the proper functioning of the immune system was overwhelmed.

The child died during her fifth day in hospital. When tests were concluded, it became apparent to doctors that Nan had become defenseless. Her young life, it seemed, had been savaged by a powerful, destructive virus: HHV-6. The autopsy suggested signs of an HHV-6 army moving unopposed through her body, attacking the heart, lungs, liver, spleen, lymph nodes, bone marrow, thymus, kidney, bladder, gastrointestinal tract, salivary glands, middle ear, peripheral nerves, and skeletal muscle. The doctors concluded in their report that Nan's death was apparently the first case of a fatal HHV-6 infection that had affected the entire body.

As researchers would discover, in the young HHV-6 could be versatile and merciless. Reports streamed in from Japan, the United States, Canada, Britain, France, Germany, Italy, and China, showing that roseola was a childhood infection that could mushroom wildly out of control. What had been first considered a mild and common childhood infection caused by a virus of seemingly modest importance was now a more complex and worrisome story.

Soon scientists realized that once HHV-6 infected children, it could cause serious problems, either sporadically or persistently, over a lifetime. HHV-6 would turn out to be a chameleon that appeared to bury itself harmlessly in the body after causing a transient infection. In time, under the right conditions, it could then explode.

New clues also began to emerge about how the virus behaved in the body over the long term. Scientists already knew that once a virus infects its host, it can become neutralized by the host's immune system and then can live harmlessly in the body until the immune system holding the virus in check is weakened. The slumbering microbe can then awaken, a process known to microbiologists as reactivation. When this occurs, viral particles can either attack the host by attaching to specific target cells or be shed from their safe niche in the body, such as the salivary glands or nerve cells, and transported through the body and expelled in body fluids and transmitted to other individuals.

Common herpes viruses are classic examples of reactivating viruses. One example is varicella zoster, the herpes virus that causes chicken pox. Once you've had the disease, you won't get it again, but the virus stays in the body and can reactivate many years later in some people to cause shingles, a painful and often scarring nerve disease. In the case of herpes virus simplex, which can cause cold sores, the virus can reactivate to cause cold sores again and again.

Scientists familiar with herpes viruses were not surprised to discover that HHV-6 was also capable of being reactivated. For example, a team of Japanese researchers, including Yamanishi, discovered that in some children who initially developed seizures when first infected, HHV-6 then burrowed its way into nerve cells, remained there dormant for several years, only to flare to life and cause more seizures.

When such research news made the scientific rounds in the late 1980s, it did not cause much of a ripple. The disease that mattered most at the time was AIDS. Many were confident that in just a few years, the unexpected monstrosity said to be caused by HIV would be put to rest with powerful treatments and even a vaccine, and then public health could return to the real war it faced: chronic lifestyle-based diseases.

The pursuit of scientific understanding is sometimes seen more as a pursuit of getting money to conduct research. While the trend toward research funding was directed primarily at lifestyle-based diseases, there were warnings from many biologists that infectious diseases, contrary to widespread belief, were not to be vanquished so easily. They pointed out that humans have had a long, dynamic relationship with the teeming hordes of viruses, bacteria, and other microbes that inhabit the planet.

At any time, a new virus somewhere on Earth can jump from animals to humans. The virus can go on a rampage because humans have not built up defenses against it. When this happens, it is called an epidemic. In the aftermath of such an event, those who were infected but survived usually are left with stronger immune systems to resist further infection from the same virus. When this process, known as immunity, occurs on a wide scale in a given population, the virus is said to be endemic, or native to that group. Eventually it becomes a routine and usually low-grade childhood infection. As times goes on, the virus and the human immune system continue to adapt to one another and arrive at a stand-off. The virus finds a safe niche in a particular organ or tissue and becomes part of human cells. Reaching this stage of symbiosis or cooperation can take millions of years. This appears to be what occurred with retroviruses, some of whose sequences have become part of the human genome.

Some biologists view cooperation as the driving force of evolution on this planet. Simple life forms merge and eventually form more complex life forms. In this light, as odd as it may seem, an infectious disease can be seen as fundamental to human life, representing a rung on the ladder to a more complex and peaceful coexistence.

Public health initiatives help pave the long road to such a cooperative state by containing the spread of microbes outside of certain infected populations. By cutting off access to more human hosts, they are designed to turn microbes eventually into mild-mannered, peace-loving types. Public health officials also try whenever possible to shore up human immune systems with vaccines, to both prevent initial microbial invasion and to consolidate the chances of a stand-off once the invading force has dug in.

In declaring victory in the war against the microbes, however, public health optimists grossly underestimated the variety of ways our rapidly changing world promotes and even accelerates change in our relationship with microbes. Like humans, microbes can also alter their evolutionary ways. Like humans, they can, if provoked and under the right conditions, go on the attack.

By contrast, those who issued warnings were more concerned about how environmental destruction, such as the plunder of vast tracts of rain forest in South America, would lead to disruptions in the stability achieved by humans and microbes.

Consider the case of malaria, which is caused by a parasite that is transmitted via the saliva of female anopheles mosquitoes. The parasite journeys through the bloodstream to the liver, where it matures, reproduces, and reappears in the blood to invade and kill blood cells and clog arteries. In some cases, death occurs within a few hours.

Fifty years ago, malaria wreaked havoc in the developing nations. With the increasing availability of antimalarial drugs and major initiatives to eradicate populations of mosquitoes, inroads were made against the disease in the 1950s and 1960s. But the effort was not enough to put the brakes on malaria. The public health system claimed victory prematurely, just when resistance to drugs was growing and no new drugs were available, and when ecological devastation pushed mosquito populations out of controlled areas and into new niches. Malaria now kills almost three million people worldwide every year. About 500 million become infected.

Tuberculosis is another example of premature public heath pronouncements of victory. The disease, caused by a mycobacterium that is capable of being passed (not easily but usually over time) from person to person through the air, had been dealt a strong blow due to the widespread use of effective drugs. But TB has nonetheless maintained itself in impoverished areas and crowded jails, and among homeless people and those with suppressed immune systems, such as organ-transplant, chemotherapy, and AIDS patients. The mycobacterium is also finding ways to adapt to, and resist, drugs that once kept it at bay.

Complacency about long-established infectious diseases was bad enough. Even worse was the attitude of experts who downplayed the likelihood of new plagues emerging. They were dismissive in the face of numerous warnings issued by biologists who understood that emergence of new infectious diseases was an ongoing phenomenon on Earth.

For biologists raising alarms, one concern was that rapid expansion of international air travel has enabled previously checked microbes to move anywhere with their human hosts. For example, what if the hemorrhagic-fever virus Ebola Zaire was to find new hosts in new regions? Identified in 1976, the disease is caused by Ebola filovirus and produces internal bleeding and shock in its victims. It is highly lethal, killing with about 90 percent efficiency. One of its cousins, Ebola Sudan, also identified in 1976, kills 50 percent of those it infects. Thus far, because such viruses are powerful killers, they have been contained to periodic outbreaks by the rapid identification of victims and their isolation.

A couple of hemorrhagic-fever viruses have already hitched rides with primates. In 1967 one traveled from East Africa to Marburg, Germany, infecting 31 research lab workers, killing seven. (It is now known as Marburg virus.) In 1989 a form of ebola identified in Asia, particularly in the Philippines, caused an outbreak in a Reston, Virginia, monkey quarantine facility. (This one was named Ebola Reston virus.)

Changes in international travel and in environments, however, are not modern phenomena. Large population movements and environmental disruptions have occurred throughout human history, leading to major outbreaks of infectious disease and epidemics. Plague, which killed many millions, became possible when people moved to crowded cities and came into contact with infected rats. Any time a microbe enters an unexposed population, there is likely to be trouble. This was a lesson of history many public health officials downplayed.

To be fair, no one could have predicted the likes of AIDS, which is now routinely blamed on the combination of more open human sexual behavior and easier long-distance travel. AIDS experts contend such changes resulted in easier transmission of HIV, which might never have been carried outside its native African region.

As for those public health officials who predicted that health prevention efforts should be refocused towards lifestyle-associated chronic diseases, such as heart ailments and cancer, they now must confront the current ideas and evidence that some of these diseases may actually be triggered by infections.

One case in point is that of ulcers, the disease of the stomach lining long thought to be caused by stress and stomach acid. The standard treatment has been antacid medicines. That is, until it was discovered that the bacterium helicobacter pylori, which lives on the stomach-wall lining, is responsible for the damage. Australian researchers Barry Marshall and Robin Warren endured two decades of ridicule by the medical establishment before their idea took hold. Now doctors routinely prescribe antibiotics to fight the microbe.

Fortunately for researchers exploring chronic disease–microbe connections, the scientific audience is more willing to consider some of the latest findings. For instance, the common bacterium chlamydia pneumoniae, which is spread by coughs and sneezes and is known to cause bronchitis and pneumonia, appears to have a role in clogging arteries. The Finnish researcher Pekka Saikku first documented that patients with this infection were four times more likely to develop heart disease than those not infected. A recent American study shows that antibiotic treatment helps cut down heart-related problems (as compared with a placebo group) in those patients who have already suffered a minor heart attack or have unstable angina.

Does C. pneumoniae help clog arteries by causing inflammation and enabling fatty substances to attach more easily to artery walls? Quite possibly. Also, if research at the National Institutes of Health is borne out, cytomegalovirus, one of HHV-6's family members, may be capable of boosting the process by reactivating and stimulating the production of smooth muscle cells that are known to be a key in plaque development.

In fact, human beings may be living with a wide array of diseases that have microbial components. Threats to our health may not only come from new microbes emerging in our changing environments, but there may also be ongoing wars inside our bodies involving old microbes that lead to disease.

In other words, if changing environments and changing human behavior are catalysts for microbes to evolve, what then happens to old microbes already nestled inside our bodies when human bodies change? What happens to microbes with reactivation potential such as HHV-6 when the immune systems of those bodies, for one reason or another, begin to destabilize?

VISION OF
A MARAUDER

Konnie Knox trusted her gut feelings. She was already detecting a pattern with HHV-6. It was preliminary, to be sure, but it was there, as revealing as the blood in the vials she manipulated every day in Donald Carrigan's laboratory.

Hired by Carrigan in 1987 as a medical technologist—in those days to work with him on his measles project—Knox, attractive and looking much younger than her 33 years, was slowly shedding her role as Carrigan's lab slave and working on more fulfilling assignments.

Clues about HHV-6 were accumulating. The strange case of 37-year-old Fred, who had been admitted to hospital suffering pneumonia, had given Knox and Carrigan a firsthand look at what the virus could do if unleashed in the body. Knox was struck in particular by how much of Fred's lung tissue was infested with HHV-6.

Now she was examining two other disturbing HHV-6 cases. The two bone marrow–transplant cases had enabled the lab to further test its ability to detect HHV-6. Without this know-how, both cases could easily have been misunderstood.

The harrowing case of 19-year-old David, referred to the lab by the hospital's transplant unit, reveals how insidious an HHV-6 infection can be. David was battling testicular cancer, a malignancy occurring mostly in young to middle-aged men, but one that often can be successfully treated. David's outlook, however, was fraught with additional danger. He had an enemy within his own body capable of reawakening and going on a rampage.

To fight David's cancer he needed a bone-marrow transplant. Marrow is the soft red and yellow fatty tissue of bone cavities; red bone marrow produces all our red blood cells and platelets, cells important to blood clotting. This young man's blood-cell production had slowed to a dangerous level.

Assessing the transplant options, doctors decided to use David's own marrow and cleanse it rather than search for a compatible donor. They extracted and froze the marrow and then treated it before transplantation in order to purge it of any malignant cells. It is a risky procedure; doctors worry about the drop in immunity brought on by the drugs used in transplantation. Weakened immunity means greater risk of developing an infection.

The extent of David's problems did not become apparent until after he required a second marrow infusion, about two months after the first. His first symptoms were fever, diarrhea, and interstitial pneumonia in both lungs. He was placed on a breathing machine and responded well; his lungs cleared in three weeks. But the pneumonia soon returned in full force. He died several weeks later.

Carrigan and Knox were asked to investigate. Studying the patient's cells, they soon eliminated the common herpes virus CMV as a possible cause. In its reactivated state, CMV has long been linked to the majority of serious post-transplant complications, such as interstitial pneumonia, a chronic inflammation of the lungs, and suppression of the proper functioning of the bone marrow, which in turn can lead to a variety of blood disorders.

Carrigan and Knox instead detected HHV-6 in samples of David's blood and bone marrow. The tests also showed that the marrow transplant had not worked and that HHV-6 had widely infected his lungs. Most of the cells infected by the virus were clustered in air sacs closely distributed near tissue that was inflamed, swollen, or dead. In contrast, normal lung tissue showed few, if any, HHV-6–infected cells.

The other case, of a 32-year-old woman, presented a greater challenge. It required painstaking follow-up work and careful interpretation of the data. Donna had been suffering from abnormal bone marrow with signs of a developing leukemia. She had received a marrow transplant from a carefully matched unrelated donor. About two weeks after the transplant, she developed a fever and interstitial pneumonia in both lungs. A wash of her bronchial tubes, samples of sputum, and a lung biopsy revealed HHV-6 infection. No other microbe appeared to be involved.

Within two weeks the woman's lung problems had cleared up, at least according to what could be seen on her X rays. But her fever, a sign of continued infection, persisted, and her white cell count continued to fall. Another two weeks went by before she showed signs of another infection, this time from CMV. After an antiviral drug was administered, her white cell count stabilized in just a few days. But on the eighth day of treatment, the interstitial pneumonia reappeared and affected her breathing, requiring her to be hooked up to a mechanical ventilator. Another wash of her breathing tubes again revealed an HHV-6 infection, but tests for the presence of CMV were now negative. With additional antiviral treatment, her lungs more or less stabilized even though her fever persisted.

Then her condition took a nasty turn. She developed pancytopenia, a condition marked by a considerable decline in red and white blood cells and platelets. Clearly her bone marrow was failing to adequately manufacture cellular elements of her blood. That's when Carrigan and Knox found HHV-6–infected cells in a sample of her bone marrow.

Antiviral treatment again saved her. The good news was that her lungs improved, her fever abated, and her overall white cell count stabilized. The bad news was that her T- and B-lymphocytes, white blood cells highly important to the proper functioning of the immune system, were at abnormally low levels, so much so that her immune system had been badly compromised. She succumbed several months later to an adenovirus infection.

It appeared that HHV-6, likely with help from its cousin CMV, had brought on the second bout of interstitial pneumonia, and that the HHV-6 had not given up, even when under attack from antiviral drugs. The virus had persisted and found a way to cause harm.

Unlike CMV, HHV-6 was known to attack T-4 lymphocytes, the only known herpes virus capable of doing so. Both patients had been antibody-positive to HHV-6 before transplantation. In both cases the virus was probably reactivated due to a drop in immunity and caused active infection. In addition, British scientists had demonstrated signs of reactivation of HHV-6 in liver transplant patients; researchers in Japan and Pennsylvania had done likewise in kidney transplant patients.

All these findings raised the question: Just how many easy victims were there for HHV-6 to attack?

Unlike her colorful colleague Donald Carrigan, Konnie Knox's past offered few clues to suggest her future as a viral pioneer. Born and bred in Milwaukee, as a youth Knox played piano and violin, and often dreamed of a career in music. Had it been suggested to her in her teens that she would lead a life in science, she probably would have been baffled. At the age of 15, after she moved with her family to the eastern shore of Maryland, she began finding reason to skip high school classes. She found schoolwork mind-numbing and turned to music for comfort.

She did admire her biology teacher, however. For several hours every week, she found schoolwork exciting and dynamic. In 1973, her senior year, a program at Marquette University in Milwaukee, leading to a career in laboratory technology, caught her eye. After visiting a local hospital to acquaint herself with this type of work, she figured there would likely be a job at the end of training. Four years later, she received her bachelor of science degree.

Knox did not immediately begin work as a medical technologist. She took a laboratory research job at the Medical College of Wisconsin, and for 10 years she studied everything from fungal infection to the requirements of a vaccine for syphilis. Knox's personal life also began to take shape: she married and gave birth to three children (with yet two more to arrive in due course).

In time, however, professional inertia began to seep in. The job felt like a dead end. Her colleagues seemed indifferent to the research work and were on automatic pilot. But Knox was not ready to quit science in favor of a domestic life. Even in her disappointing job, she gradually became more curious, more eager to learn, even if it meant having to learn on her own with no supervision or feedback.

Then she met Donald Carrigan, a scientist she viewed as a bit odd in personality but passionate about research on a new variant of measles virus. Carrigan needed a laboratory technologist to help him with the measles project. Given her duties as a mother, Carrigan doubted Knox would stay around very long, but he appreciated her intensity and considered her to be very bright. And because he neither had time nor inclination to baby-sit anyone in his lab, he particularly appreciated Knox's strong self-reliance. And while she didn't have a graduate degree, she did have research experience. So why not hire her, he thought, even if it was for the short term?

Knox came to work for Carrigan refreshingly free of the baggage that can cripple scientific innovation. That baggage includes a slavish loyalty to a particular theory, indebtedness to a sponsor with a stake in research results, and an all-round fear of offending anyone in a position of authority. The prevalence of small-mindedness in science is well-known. Volumes have been written about how vested economic interests and concerns about reputations have served to suppress free thinking in the sciences. Knox never had the opportunity to acquire such behavioral traits. She was also fortunate to have a boss like Carrigan, who stood his ground on scientific issues that mattered to him.

For Knox, being a free thinker meant questioning accepted wisdom in virology circles, specifically the wisdom surrounding a "ubiquitous" virus. If most humans are infected by HHV-6, the thinking went, how deadly could the virus be?

It takes a special person, working in special circumstances, to question a paradigm, which is usually defined as a dominant theoretical perspective in any given scientific field that organizes and guides theory and research. Thomas Kuhn, a philosopher of science known for his examination of how paradigms work, has said that sooner or later a paradigm disintegrates when it can no longer handle offsetting data. But, he warned, "novelty emerges with difficulty."

The stance taken by many scientists, particularly those involved in AIDS research, was that HHV-6 did not measure up to standards of how an "important" virus should behave. It was, after all, very common and apparently dormant in most people. How could it be a major threat to public health?

Consider what happened to Robert Gallo, leader of the National Cancer Institute who isolated HHV-6 in 1986. His finding could have led to sustained and well-funded research that would have forced scientists to consider alternatives to the theory—so quickly accepted—that one virus, HIV, caused AIDS. Here was a herpes virus that could destroy T-4 lymphocytes, at least in the test tube, more powerfully than HIV. The NCI lab work was also demonstrating that HIV and HHV-6 could interact to promote more effective and quicker killing of T-4s. Although Gallo made a strong effort to encourage researchers to consider the potential of HHV-6 as a possible co-factor in AIDS, he could not break down the resistance to the idea that a common virus could be such a killer.

Once when I heard Gallo review the data on HHV-6 at an international AIDS conference, I could sense the growing restlessness in the packed auditorium. The scientists from around the world wanted to hear about HIV. One AIDS researcher who viewed Luc Montagnier as the true discoverer of HIV even remarked cynically that Gallo wanted to show the world that he too could discover a virus first, even if the virus did not amount to much.

It did not help Gallo's case that he was willing to consider that HHV-6 might be linked to chronic fatigue syndrome (CFS). Sufferers from CFS complained of fatigue, headaches, recurrent sore throat and fever, swollen lymph nodes, inability to concentrate, impaired memory, and difficulty sleeping. Interestingly, they often mentioned catching what seemed to be a cold and never really recovering from it.

To skeptics—and there were many—these patients were suffering from "Yuppie Flu," the result of participating too strenuously in the rat race. In other words, if some of these people worked less hard, they would soon reconstitute their lost energy. The more immoderate critics of CFS claimed sufferers were either depressives or deadbeats sponging off family and society.

Gallo and his colleagues at NCI were open to the possibility that a virus was setting CFS in motion, though early studies on viruses such as Epstein-Barr virus were inconclusive. For example, in one study of a reported outbreak occurring between 1984 and 1985 at Lake Tahoe, Nevada, 105 of 150 patients had higher than normal antibody levels for EBV, 37 had normal levels, and 8 had no detectable levels at all.

The viral theory for CFS suffered a setback when scientists from the Centers for Disease Control in Atlanta conducted their own research in Lake Tahoe. They discounted EBV because antibody levels of other common viruses, including CMV, herpes simplex 1 and 2, and even measles turned up higher than routine in those diagnosed with the illness. That was about the extent of the medical detective work by the CDC. They didn't pursue the idea that an altered immune system can involve a number of changes in a virus-host relationship.

When Gallo's researchers collaborated with Lake Tahoe doctors and also found elevated antibody levels to HHV-6, they remained cautiously optimistic, until data rolled in indicating that HHV-6 infection was actually quite common. Gallo nonetheless wanted to pursue the challenge HHV-6 presented much more vigorously. But, as he would later confide to Don Carrigan, he was tired of getting "beaten up" on HHV-6. Also, personal problems that began to take up much of Gallo's time would hinder his investigation into the herpes virus.

The Gallo lab's interest in HHV-6 spurred modest bursts of other research activity, although no findings were dramatic enough to focus widespread attention on the virus. The scientific literature on HHV-6 within a few years of its discovery featured explorations of its possible role in mononucleosis-like illness; disorders of lymphoid tissue; and certain malignant diseases, including lymphoma and autoimmune disease (when the body reacts against its own tissues).

By and large, the findings were based on intriguing scientific work that showed how complex biological events can converge to produce disease. For example, in studies of an autoimmune disease known as Sjögren-Larsson syndrome, characterized by dry eyes and mouth, investigators theorized that certain viruses, including HHV-6, could trigger processes in the body that caused a kind of hyperactivity in a key component of the immune system (namely a B-lymphocyte, which is involved in antibody production) that would promote the likelihood of illness. While they did not catch the virus in the act, the researchers did offer a model of how a virus could, under certain genetic and environmental conditions, contribute to disease.

While scientific discussions such as these may be impenetrable to anyone without training in molecular and cell biology, nonetheless they are sobering reminders that when scientists decide to track a virus, there are tools to do so, and if the funding is available, there is a good chance of revealing some of its secrets.

When it became evident that HHV-6 infection was common, funding in the United States for research on the virus dwindled away. There was almost no government funding for HHV-6, and those still on the trail of the virus had to rely mainly on their own institutions, their lab budgets, and small grants from private organizations.

Once a mind-set in scientific research becomes ingrained, it is difficult to reverse direction. Ignored was the fact that Japanese scientists firmly established in 1988 that a common childhood disease known as roseola is caused by the common virus HHV-6. Or that some of the children under study had developed neurologic diseases, such as encephalitis, meningitis, seizures, and other problems including liver and kidney ailments, and that some even had horrifying deaths as HHV-6 savaged their bodies. Also disregarded was a team of researchers from the Medical College of Wisconsin that offered peculiar cases in which reactivated HHV-6 took advantage of weak immune systems to cause severe infection and disease. Such evidence related to HHV-6 was not nearly enough to pique scientific interest. Even when one of the secrets of the virus became more widely known in the early 1990s, the news hardly created a stir.

HHV-6 turned out to have two distinct forms: Variant A and Variant B. It had been known early on that there were differing "strains" of HHV-6—viruses that could be differentiated through molecular testing but were found to be sufficiently alike to be placed under one name. These strains then came to be classified into two groups. The findings pointed to HHV-6B as the variant that caused roseola. The human disease that HHV-6A caused was yet to be determined. The discovery, however, raised pivotal questions in the minds of those few scientists devoted to tracking the virus. Was B, in fact, the common one primarily acquired in childhood? Also, was it possible that A infected only certain adults?

Was the mystery surrounding the commonness of HHV-6 finally any closer to being resolved? And what might this mean for the understanding of AIDS, chronic fatigue syndrome, transplant-related infections and other diseases?

There was a great deal of work yet to be done. What was needed were scientists willing to strike out on their own. Fortunately, in Milwaukee the hunt was only just beginning.

A LAB TECH
STEPS FORWARD

For such a small and obscure scientific outpost, Donald Carrigan's laboratory was a highly productive beehive of research. From his first encounter with HHV-6, Carrigan had become consumed with a passion for research that surprised even himself. The urgency to understand the slumbering virus's secrets he found irresistible, something he could focus on with undivided attention.

Since Fred's case involving Legionnaire's disease, the lab had been making progress in charting some of HHV-6's behavior in bone marrow–transplant patients. Carrigan had been collaborating with the Marrow Transplant unit at the Medical College and another lab at the Children's Hospital of Wisconsin. Using a variety of laboratory measures in an ongoing study, he showed that HHV-6 had reawakened in the bodies of four of eight bone marrow–transplant patients, including 19-year-old David with testicular cancer and Donna, the 32-year-old woman who eventually died of an adenovirus infection. Both had developed interstitial pneumonia.

Suspecting that HHV-6 reactivations commonly occurred in marrow-transplant patients, Carrigan decided to examine lung specimens of those with the pneumonia who later had died. Finding the specimens in tissue banks, he studied nine. Sure enough, an examination of only one tissue block per patient showed that three of the nine were infected with HHV-6. A high number of infected cells were lymphocytes and immune scavenger cells called macrophages, which feed on the breakdown products of cells produced by immune system activity.

Contemplating the findings, Carrigan reasoned that if more lung tissue blocks had been available for each patient, he would have discovered that more of the victims had been infected with HHV-6. Since the study had also turned up CMV (cytomegalovirus) infections, he figured HHV-6 and its cousin CMV were possibly working in tandem to devastate the lungs.

Meanwhile, other clues were surfacing about the power of HHV-6 to cause damage in bone-marrow transplants. Reactivation of the virus was sometimes accompanied not only by high fever, fatigue, abnormal decrease of white blood cells, and interstitial pneumonia, but accumulating evidence also showed that HHV-6–infected marrow cells interfered with the ability of these cells to grow into the basic blood cells the body needs to survive. Direct infection of the marrow by HHV-6 was becoming more evident; it was, by far, the lab's most important finding.

Carrigan was pleased by the progress, but he was far from satisfied. There had been a dark cloud hovering over the lab, a potential storm by the name of Konnie Knox. The situation was so serious that he felt all the HHV-6 work could be for naught, and that HHV-6 might not get the attention it deserved. It was, however, his fault because he should have paid more attention to Knox's needs.

The seed of disaster had actually been planted in 1987, when Knox was hired. When she accepted Carrigan's offer, she failed to mention that she was a month pregnant, out of fear of not being hired. When she broke the news to him a month later, he found it difficult to understand why anyone would want yet another child. She now would have four. This suggested to Carrigan that she wasn't all that serious about devoting her life to a research career.

When she later had her fifth child, this view was further reinforced.

"What he didn't appreciate then was that although I enjoyed
children, it was also a way for me to fill what was, in part, an
empty life," Knox would later explain. "I wanted to do something
with my life, and I guess having children was something that I did
rather well. But I certainly wanted to do much more than have
kids."

When Carrigan picked up hints from Knox that she was not interested in simply doing grunt work on a measles project that had
become a giant bore, it didn't make a strong impression on him. "I
guess I hadn't figured her out very well," he would later admit.

"These macho type of guys don't do much thinking of women
wanting careers too," she interjected. "They only learn the hard
way."

"She's right," Carrigan said.

He was surprised when Knox, a year after starting at the lab,
began her master's degree in business management, although he
could grudgingly accept that the degree could be an important
escape hatch for the day she tired of lab work. Becoming a lab bu-
reaucrat, after all, was a common path followed by lab technolo-
gists. During Knox's two years of course work for the degree,
Carrigan allowed her to follow a flexible schedule at the lab. He
depended on her for her quality work on the bone-marrow project, but, if truth be known, he also thought it would be good to
have someone around who had the skills to manage a lab. His lab.
That would free him from some of the drudgery and the time he
needed to address the needs of graduate students who worked under his supervision.

"He thought that he'd really have a good deal if I became a lab
mother, teaching his students and making sure everything ran
smoothly," she said, laughing.

But Carrigan was wrong. He terribly misjudged Knox and now
would pay for it.

The crisis reached critical mass when Judy, a microbiology graduate student working in the lab, asked to be involved in the bone-

marrow project, not as a gofer but as Carrigan's colleague. This was not unusual, considering graduate students often end up doing some of the breakthrough research for which their advisers claim credit. Those graduate students not easily intimidated into suppressing their egos expect to receive the appropriate respect.

Carrigan considered Judy a fine lab technologist, and because she was his only grad student at the time, he gave her more attention and encouragement than he normally would have, including the opportunity to present an abstract of some of the lab's ongoing bone-marrow research at a conference on herpes viruses.

When Knox found out, she hit the roof. Her frustration had been building. At work, she was not getting the respect she felt she deserved. At home, her marriage had been rocky for months. What she needed most was a job that was worthy of her intelligence and spirit.

Knox felt that she was often coming up with new ideas for research, even if officially she was a lab techie. So what if she wasn't a microbiology grad student like Judy, heading for an academic career? Knox and Carrigan often discussed Knox's ideas and put them on the research agenda. Now here was this grad student getting the opportunity to present their scientific research to the world. She also wanted that opportunity.

"He was ignoring my accomplishments," Knox said.

She had been conducting research in the lab showing that HHV-6 could infect—and suppress—bone-marrow cells. The virus inhibited the fundamental elements of bone marrow—called precursors—that are involved in manufacturing basic blood cells. This was further evidence that HHV-6 could directly attack the marrow, and reinforced the lab's findings in the ongoing study of transplant patients. The virus appeared to be capable of disabling the complex interactive environment of the marrow by attacking cells and activating chemicals.

Such attacks on the marrow could cause a range of bad effects, from mild anemia (decreased red cell production) and fatal aplastic anemia (a deficiency in all the basic elements of blood) to hemorrhage (loss of a large amount of blood).

Carrigan certainly appreciated Knox's research, given her steadfast contribution to the lab's accumulating knowledge on HHV-6. Yet he primarily viewed her as a lab techie and not an aspiring research scientist. "I simply didn't see Konnie as being on the same career track as Judy, no matter how Konnie excelled at innovative research," Carrigan said sheepishly. "Yeah, I was blind to it."

"I finally let him have it," Knox said. "You might say that it was a blistering attack, and it stunned him."

Carrigan didn't know what he was going to do to preserve the peace. He didn't want to lose the best lab technologist he'd ever had. There was no denying he enjoyed her quick wit. Sometimes she was even a good pal. He left his meeting with Knox shaken. Had he turned out to be the type of a scientist he had always hated—the paternalist who couldn't accord the women he worked with the same respect as a male colleague?

As part of his damage-control strategy, Carrigan decided to subsidize a trip for Knox to attend an academic meeting so that she could present some of the laboratory results on HHV-6 suppression of bone marrow. But tension between Knox and Judy still existed. They worked in close proximity in a small lab. How long could they continue to work together? Perhaps he could hold planning meetings with them separately, in his office and in the cafeteria, to help diffuse outright competition. He knew one thing: he was tired of having to worry about the situation. There was exciting and important research to perform. That had to take priority over all else.

Early one morning in August 1991, Konnie Knox announced to Donald Carrigan that she wanted to attend graduate school at Medical College and earn her Ph.D. She told Carrigan that her mind was made up and that she wanted him to be her doctoral adviser. If he did not accept, she would find someone else.

Knox was at a turning point in her life. She was 37 years old and her marriage had just ended. She was acutely aware of—and frustrated by—the limitations of her scientific knowledge. But in choosing to upgrade her education, Knox was being entirely pragmatic: not having those arcane letters of Ph.D. after her name had become a curse. If she wanted respect as a researcher, a doctorate would be essential. The confrontation with Carrigan over her role in the lab had convinced her of that. Even Donald Carrigan, despite his independent nature, had not realized a technologist would want recognition.

Knox did not expect Carrigan's reaction. "He went rigid like a block of stone," she said. Later he would confess to her that his "unfriendly" reaction was "knee-jerk" and "unfair." At the time he was emotionally drained and could not imagine where he would find the time to, in his words, "baby-sit" yet another graduate student. But by the time blood flow returned to his face, he was already considering the possibility that she might not qualify for entrance into graduate school because of insufficient preparatory course work. "I didn't expect her to be accepted," he said, "but I agreed to become her adviser-in-waiting."

Knox had her own concerns. As an undergraduate, she had been only an average student and had never scored high in college admissions tests. Yet she was not prepared for the blatant sexism she experienced during interviews for admission to the graduate school. More than one department chair suggested that someone of her age who had five children should not even think about returning to school. She was advised to go home and take care of her family.

And, as Carrigan anticipated, her academic reviewers found fault with her qualifications. They especially emphasized her lack of adequate preparation in biochemistry. Knox fought back, gamely proposing to enroll in that one biochemistry course at Medical College, with the understanding that if she passed it with flying colors, her application would be accepted. After hemming and hawing, a deal was struck. She would begin the course in January 1992, and aim to complete her requirements by June.

Carrigan was furious at his colleagues at Medical College. "I couldn't believe that they would give her such a hard time," he said, adding that the shameful exhibition of academic arrogance also fueled his own guilt concerning the way he had behaved toward her. He was now realizing that he would need to adapt even more to Knox's needs if he wished to have a sound working relationship with her. Since it had been 16 years since he took a biochemistry course, he went so far as to buy the required text-book for himself, in case she needed help with her course assignments. Carrigan also decided that he would give Knox flexible lab hours so that she could tend to school and family. Should her children become ill, for example, he would even pick up some of the slack by helping out with her lab duties. Only with the benefit of hindsight would Carrigan come to see that, in making such personal accommodations, he effectively ensured that research in the lab would continue to unmask HHV-6.

Several months into the biochemistry course, Knox felt Carrigan had come to appreciate her more as an equal. "He gave me the impression that he was trying very hard," she said. They shared information on biochemistry and interacted far more extensively on research plans. In so doing, they also revealed more of their differences.

Carrigan was a highly conservative scientist, not given to intuitive leaps. He wanted to see detailed, reliable data before he became confident they were on the right track. In contrast, Knox was always pushing him to perceive patterns that projected beyond the available data. For example, she was already beginning to set her sights on research that would explore the role HHV-6 played in AIDS. Since the NCI lab data had shown that HIV and HHV-6 could work together, she was certain the same would hold true in the body. Since HHV-6 was so common, could it reactivate in people whose immune systems were depleted? Of course it could. Why would the virus not take advantage? While Carrigan was intrigued by Knox's theories, he was uncomfortable with ideas that ranged so far ahead of expected scientific reasoning.

It had occurred to Knox more than once that Carrigan might lack the ability to think big. It certainly had occurred to Carrigan that Knox might be too undisciplined to take one research step at a time. After some discussion Carrigan came away thinking it was pointless to argue with Knox on certain matters; she believed she saw things clearly, even if the science was in the preliminary stage. For her part, Knox left their meetings wondering how much caution she was willing to endure.

As for Judy, with her graduate studies ending, she was less

involved with the HHV-6 research. During her stay she had
contributed her fair share to the investigation, which was now
broadening. For example, one study that tracked 16 bone marrow–
transplant patients for several months showed further evidence
of marrow suppression by HHV-6 after transplantation. By this
time Carrigan and Knox were beginning to differentiate between
HHV-6A and HHV-6B infection, due to new testing materials that
other labs had made available. This study showed reactivation of
HHV-6B, the strain associated with roseola.

While Carrigan and Knox were intrigued by the evidence that
HHV-6 was divided into two distinct variants, the issue would take
on importance in their work only gradually. They had too many
other details they hoped to unearth about HHV-6 before they
would decide to focus more of their time on the strategies the virus
was using to maintain an advantage over its human targets.

One key issue on their agenda was to determine how HHV-6
damaged the ability of bone marrow to manufacture basic blood
cells. Carrigan and Knox already determined that the virus appeared capable of accomplishing this feat. They theorized that,
among other possibilities, the virus, in attacking the marrow, could
inhibit a chemical called a "growth factor" that normally assists in
the blood-production process. A new study in the lab supported
the hypothesis. The study showed that when the virus (both A and
B variants) interferes with growth factors, it can block production
of macrophages, vital immune cells that mop up microbes and cellular debris.

Carrigan and Knox were troubled by the immediate implications of their findings. In medicine it was common to use growth
factors as therapy to help support a bone-marrow transplant and
to fight off marrow suppression in cancer victims. They considered
it probable that HHV-6 infection was the cause of some of the reported poor responses to this type of therapy in such patients.

On another front, Carrigan had worked with Judy to show that
HHV-6 affected the normal functions of an important immune cell
called a monocyte, the largest white cell found in blood. Like a
macrophage, it too ingests and disposes of microorganisms and
cellular debris. If its internal signals are disturbed, as the research

revealed, this could potentially lead in some patients to further immune suppression and weakened defense against bacterial, fungal, and viral infections. In such a case, the researchers noted, HHV-6A appeared to be better than HHV-6B at sabotaging monocytes.

To Carrigan, the research was edging closer to pinning down the possible ways that HHV-6 crippled bone marrow. He believed further refinements would result in an understanding of the infection process, and that could save the lives of many thousands of patients. This would take hard work and huge amounts of time, but he was deeply committed to the research path, one that he pioneered.

Knox had other ideas.

In May 1992, when Knox completed her biochemistry course with a B-plus grade, Medical College accepted her into graduate school.

Her big question was what to focus on. The power of HHV-6 to menace bone marrow was Carrigan's domain; she needed a different area. AIDS seemed an excellent candidate, and not because it had the highest profile among medical scientists. Knox was fascinated by how HHV-6, like HIV, attacked T-4 lymphocytes, monocytes, and macrophages.

Knox was aware of the controversies raging around HIV. Scientists were not sure how the virus destroyed the immune system. Some, a vocal minority, were convinced that HIV, the so-called "AIDS virus," could not possibly cause AIDS. One of the dissidents, Peter Duesberg, had referred to HIV as a "pussycat." But there was little serious consideration being given to any causal factor in AIDS other than HIV, which Knox felt was another reason for her to be a trailblazer. On the other hand, by focusing on the role of HHV-6 in AIDS for her doctoral thesis, Knox wondered, was she throwing herself into the hurly-burly of Big Science politics?

THE CONTROVERSY
IN AIDS RAGED ON

"Welcome to the bunker." Peter Duesberg offered a disarmingly warm smile with the sardonic greeting as he led the way into his University of California laboratory. For a man whose face often sported a boxer's glare, Duesberg appeared surprisingly delicate and subdued. "So, have you seen my old friend Big Bob being chased by all those investigators?" he asked. Duesberg was referring to an NIH investigation of Gallo's early claims for the discovery of HIV. "Maybe he should come to Berkeley and live in the bunker with me, his old friend Duesberg."

"No, I haven't seen him in a while," I replied, knowing the comment was ironic. I had a flashback to 1987, to a going-away party for Duesberg at the NIH. Duesberg's year-long stint at the NIH was ending, and his colleagues were wining and dining him. But the one person missing at the party was Gallo. Duesberg wanted to know why he didn't show and so he telephoned Gallo, then reported back to the group, "Big Bob has again refused to date me."

The past several years had not been a good time for Gallo. After a seven-year battle with the United States government, the Pasteur Institute had wrested away most of the credit for the discovery of HIV. In May 1991, a humbled Gallo had to admit in a letter to the journal *Nature* that his virus, HTLV-3, was somehow the product of a laboratory mix-up with the French virus, LAV.

Duesberg was not exactly broken up by Gallo's misfortune. In the past few years Duesberg had endured professional trauma of his own: criticism in medical journals; cancelled media interviews at the last minute due to pressure tactics from scientists, including those in the government; and roadblocks to getting his scientific papers published. The latest insult—and perhaps the most troublesome to stomach—was the non-renewal by the NIH of his $350,000-per-year "outstanding investigator research grant." The two labs that made up his unit were in danger of being closed due to the funding cut. At the same time, the university would no longer allow him to teach graduate students.

"They tell me that I have spent too much time criticizing AIDS research," he said with bitterness. "They say that even though I am a pioneer in retrovirology, I am becoming too unproductive, I'm no longer at the top of my field. They refuse to accept that I'm being productive in challenging the kind of retrovirology that is making this huge AIDS mistake." Punitive? Absolutely. "This is one way science tells you that you are dead," he said. Take aim at the establishment once too often and pay the price of your convictions. Duesberg had anticipated getting shunned for his view that HIV does not cause AIDS, but he had not expected to lose his career grant, the core of his enterprise.

Close to a decade of AIDS research, focused almost entirely on HIV, had passed and several billions of dollars had been spent worldwide to fight and prevent the syndrome, yet there was no cure, no vaccine, and only highly risky and controversial antiviral treatment.

Meanwhile, still unproven and often complex theories about how AIDS devastated the body's immune system were multiplying. Some scientists were trying to account for the death of immune cells even a decade after initial HIV infection. They were studying the possibility that the body's lymph nodes could trap HIV in certain cells. When these cells broke down, they would supposedly eject a burst of HIV particles into the bloodstream.

AIDS researchers were building even more elaborate hypotheses, suggesting that a combination of invasions by HIV, other infections, and perhaps drug abuse was tricking the immune system into attacking itself. This was one form of the AIDS "autoimmune" theories making the scientific rounds, yet there still was no compelling autoimmune evidence.

In short, many avenues were being explored to show how clever and complex HIV was in dismantling the immune system. There were so many avenues, in fact, that a growing number of scientists began thinking of a co-factor theory, the idea that some other factor, such as a virus or bacterium, helped HIV do its work.

The most intriguing development came not from the AIDS establishment but from the maverick research of Shyh-Ching Lo, an inquisitive scientist at the fortress-like Armed Forces Institute of Pathology in Washington, D.C. The institute is one of the world's most reputable and highly specialized centers for research on dead tissue. Lo's work, and how it fit into the sprawling AIDS research environment, offered a rare insight into the politically charged behavior of the times.

Lo had never been convinced that HIV was the killer of T-4 lymphocytes and therefore the sole cause of AIDS. Whenever he investigated a tissue sample from someone who had died of AIDS, he did not find evidence of HIV-inflicted damage. "If there is no sign of the virus in the diseased tissue, it should raise some questions," he said. "It made me suspicious and made me look harder at the tissue."

While he could not find HIV, he did find evidence of a microbe that he referred to as a "virus-like infectious agent," or VLIA. The agent turned up in mice cells he injected with tissue from the spleen of one man who had died of AIDS and with Kaposi's sarcoma tissue from another AIDS fatality. He then developed a test from isolates of the new agent to detect signs of it in blood indirectly. In one study of 24 people with AIDS, 23 tested positive for the agent. His findings were first published in a niche-market tropical disease journal because no mainstream science periodical accepted it. When Lo presented his work in 1988 at the Fourth International AIDS Conference in Stockholm, he was given the cold shoulder.

Not long after the conference, I asked Gallo for his opinion of Lo's work. Twisting in his office seat at the NCI, he said, "Who in the hell is this guy anyway? What has been proved? Absolutely nothing. It's probably a bunch of crap."

In April 1989, Lo published more detailed findings. In seven of 10 people with AIDS, he found signs of VLIA in the spleen, liver, brain, and lymph nodes. There was no sign of the agent in people without AIDS. He concluded cautiously: "Our findings suggest that VLIA may represent a new opportunistic infection in these severely immunocompromised patients, or an agent that plays a more fundamental role as a co-factor in the process associated with infection by HIV."

In questioning the role played by HIV, this research, finally, attracted the attention of the AIDS establishment. Critics let loose a barrage. VLIA was probably a lab error, a contaminant. Why was Lo not sharing his molecular materials on the virus with the rest of the scientific world? Why was the army allowing him to be so secretive? What was he hiding?

Gallo wanted to do the testing himself. He sent Lo a letter requesting the molecular probes for VLIA but was rebuffed. The institute would release them only to a handful of researchers who had entered collaborative agreements, and the institute refused even to identify who the scientists were. Gallo commented, "What they are doing borders on the criminal."

Had his opinion on HIV changed? Well, not really. "Maybe it's a contaminant," he said at the time. "Or it could be a miscellaneous pathogen that can cause disease in some people but is not involved in causing immune suppression."

Some scientists, however, were concerned about Gallo's antics. Norbert Rapoza, a virologist and senior scientist at the American Medical Association, speculated ominously that should the army consent to NCI involvement, "Gallo with his army of researchers would devour Lo."

In September 1989, Lo published again, showing that VLIA could be lethal. He linked the agent to six deaths associated with an infectious disease without a definable cause. The pathological specimens from these cases showed no sign of HIV. The six people had died within seven weeks after flu-like symptoms were reported to their doctors. The deaths were then reported to the institute by pathologists in New Jersey, Virginia, Florida, Germany, Turkey, and Guam. Shared symptoms included persistent fever, malaise, vomiting, diarrhea, and aching joints and muscles.

The course of the disease varied. For example, one 29-year-old man, previously healthy according to his medical charts, developed symptoms in the following sequence: knee pain, sensitivity to light, blurred vision, eye infection, fever without chills, pain in the ankles, elbows, and hips, a dry cough, breathing difficulty on exertion, chest pain, lesions in his lungs, a spleen abnormality. At the end, he died of a heart attack. A previously healthy 33-year-old woman suffered from fever, chills, enlarged lymph nodes, diarrhea, vomiting, a skin rash, nausea, malaise, seizures, a chest disorder, and kidney failure.

When Lo examined the pathological specimens, he found signs of VLIA and particles resembling it in areas of excessive tissue damage. There were no signs in the diseased tissue of other viruses, bacteria, fungi, or parasites. He expected to find signs of strong immune-system reaction to the invasion of the tissue but did not. He concluded that either the body's defense system was damaged or VLIA somehow eluded it.

With further laboratory research Lo finally identified VLIA as a novel mycoplasma—a bacterium-like ultramicroscopic organism and cousin to one that was known to cause pneumonia, inflammation of the windpipe, and breathing tubes, as well as other infections. VLIA, which Lo renamed Mycoplasma incognitus, also turned out to interest Luc Montagnier, who believed a possible co-factor in AIDS might turn up. In March 1990, Montagnier shocked many HIV researchers when he released the results of an unusually simple study in the Pasteur Institute journal *Research in Virology*. He demonstrated that cultured cells with HIV, when given the antibiotic tetracycline, grew well, when usually they died quickly without the antibiotic. The treatment could not possibly have affected HIV since antibiotics do not kill viruses, so Montagnier assumed some undetected bacterium had been killing the cells. He deduced that mycoplasma might be the villain because they typically invade cell cultures. He was particularly impressed with Lo's findings and believed it was plausible that incognitus behaved as an AIDS co-factor.

Three months later, in San Francisco at the Sixth International Conference on AIDS, Montagnier spoke about his latest investigation. Yet what he thought would be watershed news was instead greeted by heckles and guffaws. The discoverer of the "AIDS virus" was, in the eyes of his detractors, going off the deep end.

Gallo, meanwhile, stood his ground. He had been trying, with considerable difficulty, to make the case that HHV-6 could boost HIV's attack on the immune system. But unlike Montagnier, who was now willing to consider the possibility that HIV, while necessary, might be insufficient to cause AIDS, Gallo said that he was convinced that HIV was all that was required. HHV-6 only added to the power of HIV. He felt that Montagnier had broken ranks. What a boon this was for Peter Duesberg, who was waiting for someone in the mainstream to concede that HIV was only part of the story.

Gallo read Peter Duesberg accurately. Duesberg believed that when microbiologists begin looking for co-factors, it suggests that they are confused about the cause of a disease. To Duesberg, this latest chapter in AIDS research showed the uncertain foundation upon which HIV theory was based. If Montagnier thought that a co-factor might be necessary for AIDS to develop, then it meant that a sea change could be occurring in mainstream thinking.

Duesberg had his own theory about what caused AIDS. According to him, toxic factors, not infectious ones, destroyed the immune system. In most AIDS cases the body was laid waste by a host of infections that went wild once the immune system had been ravaged by long-term and cumulative intake of intravenous, recreational, and pharmaceutical drugs, notably the toxic anti-HIV drug AZT. "People do not realize how much drugs people with

AIDS have typically consumed, and the ability of numerous recreational drugs to damage immunity," Duesberg said. "These drugs,
such as cocaine, amphetamines, intravenous drugs, and nitrite in-
halants often used by homosexuals to have more sex fun cause
classic AIDS symptoms." He emphasized that AZT, the first antiviral approved for AIDS, was highly toxic to cells, a fact essentially spelled out in official descriptions of the drug. AZT was
originally developed to kill cancer cells by interrupting their ability to synthesize DNA. Duesberg believed that many HIV-positive
people who were quickly prescribed AZT would not have developed AIDS had they steered clear of this "poison."

On the basis of an extensive review of the scientific literature,
Duesberg published a lengthy article linking AIDS to the huge
jump in the overall use of drugs, particularly since the early 1970s
among some groups particularly vulnerable to the syndrome, notably gay men and intravenous drug users. He also argued that
non-infectious immune-suppressant factors in blood transfusions
could lead to AIDS, as could injections of factor 8, a potentially
immune-damaging coagulation substance present in normal plasma
taken by hemophiliacs.

Duesberg did not expect Bob Gallo and the HIV establishment
to take his scholarship seriously. And now that he had published
details of his theory, he would have to assess how he could continue to survive in his lab at Berkeley without the renewal of his
career grant. But he vowed not to throw in the towel. Sooner or
later, he predicted, more evidence would appear that would force
the HIV theory to capsize.

What Duesberg didn't know was that a graduate student in
Milwaukee was about to enter the fray with new data on a herpes
virus, one that might, under certain conditions, kill T-4 lymphocytes in the body and not only in the lab.

FLESHING OUT A STRANGER WITHIN

The 34 autopsy samples harvested from nine people who had died of AIDS were sent from a Milwaukee hospital to the Carrigan lab "fixed" in formalin, a disinfectant and preservative for biological specimens, and embedded in paraffin. Soon after the package arrived in the summer of 1993, Konnie Knox eagerly yet meticulously analyzed each sample by drawing on elaborate procedures that determine whether or not a viral infection is active at the time of death.

In this first phase of her doctoral project since being admitted to graduate school, Knox was expecting to find evidence that HHV-6 played a role in the development of AIDS. It was turning out that the virus could be awakened in people with immune-system defects. It stood to reason the same would apply among AIDS patients. But she did not anticipate just how much HHV-6 infection she would find.

The results of her experiments gave her a jolt: all 34 tissue samples of lung, lymph node, liver, kidney, and spleen revealed that at the time of death there was active HHV-6 infection, as opposed to merely a biological sign that the virus was "latent" (embedded in the tissue). Since these tissue types had been provided for almost all the cases, Knox was also able to determine that the active infection had become widespread. This was significant because CMV, HHV-6's closest herpes virus family member, was generally considered to be one of the most common infections to arise in people with AIDS once their immune systems became crippled. Knox's experiments showed that only nine of 34 tissue samples had been infected with CMV. Since she had not preselected the tissue she had studied, it was possible that the pattern she had unearthed could be common.

Knox was particularly struck by the magnitude of HHV-6 lung-infected tissue. HHV-6 had attacked the lungs of all nine of the deceased. In one of the six patients who had died from respiratory failure, the density of HHV-6 infection was so great that she suspected the virus was directly to blame. Previously, the cause of this patient's lung disease had not been diagnosed. Here was a likely example of how the virus could cause lethal organ damage in someone with AIDS.

The lymph node tissue that Knox studied provided her with more food for thought. Tissue samples from five of six patients revealed that HHV-6 had infected few cells, mostly debris-devouring macrophages. For the most part, other than show that the virus could enter the tissue, it was not clear what was responsible for the depletion of other types of cells, particularly lymphocytes. The common—and still contentious—view was that HIV somehow had killed the cells.

Tissue from the sixth patient offered Knox an important clue. The node was highly infected with HHV-6, and mostly so in the lymphocytes in one particular region. It turned out that the patient, unlike the others whose tissues had been collected, had died early from a rare pneumonia. Did this mean that HHV-6 plundered lymphocytes in lymph nodes early in the AIDS process? If so, how early? Knox vowed to find out.

She did not have the field entirely to herself. In November 1993, Robert Gallo's lab published data gleaned from autopsies of five people who had died of AIDS, demonstrating an abundance of HHV-6 infection. Footprints of the virus were found in areas such as the cerebral cortex, brain stem, cerebellum, spinal cord, tonsil, lymph nodes, spleen, bone marrow, salivary glands, esophagus, bronchial tree, lung, skeletal muscle, myocardium, aorta, liver, kidney, adrenal glands, pancreas, and thyroid. The difference between the NCI study and Knox's was that the government scientists had not shown "active" infection at the time of death. The lab tools they used to detect gene sequences of HHV-6 were not sensitive enough to set apart an active from a latent infection. Because of the widespread infection uncovered at NCI, however, they assumed that the infection was active. Nonetheless, Knox the grad student had beaten the big guys to the punch, and she naturally wondered why research of this type had not previously been conducted by AIDS researchers, considering that Gallo had strongly proposed that HHV-6 was a co-factor in AIDS. "I was really amazed that so little HHV-6 research had actually been done on AIDS patients," she later said. "It didn't make much sense."

Gallo and his colleagues continued to regard HHV-6 as a potential accelerator or "catalyst" of HIV infection and progression to AIDS. They viewed their own study and Knox's as more proof of this co-factor vision. But until a long-term study carefully tracked how HHV-6 was linked to the AIDS process, doubts would remain about its importance.

That certainly was one way of thinking about HHV-6, though it was not Knox's way. But considering what had been going on behind the scenes involving Carrigan, Knox was fortunate to even have the opportunity to continue her AIDS research.

Knox came close to not starting her graduate program as scheduled, at least not with Carrigan as her thesis adviser. For several months before she started the AIDS project, Carrigan had been having a tough time with one of his superiors at Medical College. Carrigan felt he was being pushed too hard to mentor some of the junior faculty, as he had been expected to do. "I figured he might be envious of the attention that our lab was receiving because of the numerous publications coming out," Carrigan explained. "So one day I blew my stack and said some harsh things, and of course, he advised that he would take steps to fire me for insubordination."

Knox was concerned about losing a colleague she increasingly valued and admired. But when he hinted of receiving job offers, she became panic-stricken about losing her thesis adviser. All the effort that had gone into building a mutually respectful relationship was about to go down the drain.

"When I went to see the enemy to give my support to Don, he suggested that he become my adviser," Knox recalled. "Don was horrified at the prospect and immediately groveled for forgiveness, promising him that he would mentor the junior faculty."

"I only wanted to get him off my back," Carrigan said.

It was to be a short-lived peace. Carrigan admitted he had neither the head for the politics of science nor the time to think about it. "You know what?" he asked. "I just don't give a shit."

Instead he continued to concentrate on tracking HHV-6. Both he and Knox were beginning to understand just how efficiently the virus makes a home for itself in the human body, and how nasty it could become when disturbed.

The fact that HHV-6 had existed for a long time was one indication that the virus had developed effective—and sustainable—evolutionary strategies. Critical to its survival is only lightly infecting most individuals before becoming dormant. If it destroyed its host, where would it live? Being a parasite, it cannot survive on its own. Still, HHV-6 maintains enough of its firepower to protect itself should there be any change in the relationship with its host's immune system.

Carrigan and Knox came to suspect that HHV-6 was highly aggressive, always pushing against an immune system that was keeping it in check. They believed that once there was even a mild drop in the immune system's hold on the virus, the peace could give way to a renewed attack. Obeying a certain grim biological logic, the virus would multiply and attack body cells at any lessening release of the body's immunological restraints. When most of these flare-ups occurred, it seemed, only a mild infection would develop, followed by another truce. In some cases, however, HHV-6 could cause more widespread infection. And when the immune system suffered a severe blow, as Carrigan and Knox observed, HHV-6 would rampage. In their laboratory experiments and in studies of seriously ill patients, they noticed that a severe drop in immunity appeared to transform HHV-6 into a killer.

The virus also seemed capable of disabling key components of the immune system itself. When the Gallo lab isolated the virus in 1986, the NCI scientists believed HHV-6 mostly caused infection in B-lymphocytes—white blood cells that are key soldiers in the immune system army. It is their job to seek out, identify and, through the production of antibodies, bind to molecular patterns or "receptors" that sit on the surface of cells or toxic molecules. Normally they play a significant role in knocking foreign invaders out of commission.

While HHV-6 did indeed attack some B-cells, further studies at NCI showed the virus was mostly interested in attacking T-4 lymphocytes, another of the immune system's key soldiers. Unlike B-cells, T-4-cells do not produce antibodies, but instead travel and bind to cells seen as foreign or abnormal and then release chemicals that help destroy the invaders.

Various laboratories exposed HHV-6 as capable of targeting other immune cells, including T-8 lymphocytes, and of disabling the proper maturation, function, or effectiveness of scavenger cells that mop up infected cells and the war-produced debris in the blood. In addition, Carrigan and Knox had already showed that the virus could attack bone marrow.

The culmination of these efforts came in April 1993, when scientists at NCI demonstrated in the laboratory that HHV-6 infects and kills natural killer cells. These are the immune cells that destroy abnormal cells in the body, particularly those that are infected by viruses. HHV-6 is the first virus known to be capable of targeting and seriously damaging such a vital element of the immune system's antiviral defenses.

In both the Gallo and Carrigan labs, it did not escape notice that natural killer cell function is, in varying degrees, disabled in both AIDS and chronic fatigue syndrome patients. Gallo and his colleagues again proposed—as they had been doing repeatedly since learning how efficiently HHV-6 killed T-4 cells—that studies in humans could show how HHV-6 contributed to the immune problems seen in both AIDS and CFS. While committed to exploring that path, which proposed HHV-6 as a player in both syndromes, Carrigan and Knox were about to raise the virus's profile another level entirely.

Though they were working together, that did not mean they were always in harmony. As they argued over how to proceed, the raised voices in the Carrigan lab could be heard by researchers working all the way down the hall. As a natural outgrowth of the tedious and repetitive work of a modern laboratory, frustrations and time pressures often lead to emotional outbursts. It is expected and accepted, within reason. But in the case of the two intense HHV-6 researchers, the fights had been becoming more frequent ever since Knox had become a graduate student.

Carrigan had agreed that Knox would be responsible for her own project. She would focus most of her attention on AIDS and assist him on ongoing bone marrow–transplant studies and any of the medical mysteries local clinicians brought to their attention. In turn, he would collaborate on the AIDS research as an adviser and assist her in writing scientific papers. That was the plan. Only these days, by the fall of 1993, a shrill Knox was accusing Carrigan of interfering with her research. She was particularly upset about his coming in some mornings and performing preparatory lab work without her permission. He had his bone marrow–transplant pioneering, Knox figured, so why could he not get it into his head that she wanted to chart something herself? It was her doctoral degree, after all.

"On one level, I thought it was cool that Don was interested in my work, that he recognized the importance of the project. But I had to insist that whenever I worked on AIDS, he would have to butt out of the lab and leave me in peace."

For his part, the spurned Carrigan wondered why Knox could not see that he was only trying to be helpful. She had a monster schedule, being a single mother to five kids, as well as a full-time graduate student.

"Konnie never fully appreciated the pressures of her own time constraints. She survived her various crises because people were helping her. Even her former husband came around to her home

and took care of the kids. Her mother helped as well. Charles
Darwin would have loved her: here was a terrific survivor, carefully selecting people to play certain roles in her life so that she
could achieve what she wanted."

Still, during this difficult period of adjustment, Knox managed
to stay remarkably focused on her AIDS project. It always as-
tounded Carrigan that she could fix her attention on her lab work
so intently. His theory was that she had learned to spare her energy
and largely avoided people who she assessed were peripheral to
her interests. He, on the other hand, could not compartmentalize
his emotions and sometimes found it difficult to keep his mind on
work. This was especially true now, as his bureaucratic nemesis
continued to hound him to help junior faculty with their research.
Carrigan was a scientist, not a glorified baby-sitter.

Knox knew Carrigan was under the gun but figured he would
weather the storm as he had on previous occasions. When push
came to shove, Carrigan would try to smooth out the situation by
making minor concessions and then resort to his carefully plotted
avoidance tactics. Anyway, Knox thought, Medical College would
not mess with a scientist as productive as Carrigan, who was
becoming a star on campus. The publication output on bone
marrow–transplants and HHV-6 was impressive, and there was
more to come, including her research on AIDS.

Knox sensed that she could break new ground in showing how
HHV-6 behaved in AIDS patients. She knew that the virus was extremely active at the time of their deaths. She also had learned it
could cause major damage to lymph nodes during the early development of AIDS. Now she wanted to know how early such damage occurred. Could it be even before AIDS was diagnosed? That
would be an eye opener—an unheralded virus causing damage
usually considered the sole handiwork of HIV. But such a finding
would not come as a shock to Knox, considering the nodes were
loaded with lymphocytes, the chief targets of HHV-6.

Laboratory research is mostly grunt work. The days can be
long and uninspiring; traveling from point A to B en route to Z
typically requires the performance of many hours of monotonous

and meticulous tasks. It can only be hoped that each step in the process leads without error to the next. Researchers try to come up with antidotes to the humdrum: presenting ongoing work at a scientific forum; discussing results of recent experiments with television or newspaper reporters; basking in the energy derived from a true and budding friendship; or experiencing the pure excitement that discovery brings.

For Carrigan and Knox, a combination of all of the above gave them the required energy to get on with the obligatory tasks. Additionally, colleagues from hospitals associated with Medical College would refer mystery medical cases to them, hoping they could unravel them. This type of problem file got their juices flowing even more, since it helped them explore HHV-6. The Legionnaire's disease case referred to Carrigan in 1988 had set the wheels in motion. The transplant unit at Medical College had provided Carrigan and Knox with numerous opportunities to study HHV-6 in bone marrow–transplant patients. And now doctors from Children's Hospital of Wisconsin provided them with a case that would open a new door.

This time the patient was Marie, a young child whose life was dramatically snuffed out a little more than a year after she entered the world. Life had begun badly for Marie. The Milwaukee infant weighed less than six pounds, her body temperature fluctuated, and she had difficulty feeding. The baby had to remain in the hospital for five days before she was considered stable enough to be discharged.

Once home, Marie still fussed at feeding time. At four months old, she took a turn for the worse, landing in the hospital with a fever and requiring oxygen because of a respiratory infection. Tests identified the herpes virus CMV as well as Pneumocystis carinii, a bacterium that can infect the lungs when the immune system is overwhelmed. Its presence is considered the calling card of AIDS, but there was no sign of HIV. Marie's lymphocyte count, however, was abnormally low, and her thymus gland, which essentially conditions lymphocytes to become T-cells and to protect the immune system against infections, was abnormally small. Even though these were signs of serious immune damage, her doctors concluded that drug therapy administered intravenously was the only available practical strategy. After eight long, trying weeks in the hospital, the six-month-old child was discharged.

At eight months of age, Marie continued to lose weight, despite receiving high-caloric feedings through a special tube. Once again she was briefly admitted to the hospital for observation. Once again, doctors clung to drug therapy as the child's only hope of recovery.

At 13 months, there were more signs of impending doom: continued weight loss and more serious breathing problems. Marie was readmitted. In an effort to help her breathe, a tube was placed in her trachea, and she was hooked up to a mechanical ventilator. Marie's lungs continued to show signs of CMV and P. carinii, and despite more drug treatments, her immune system was no stronger. The youngster died in the hospital of lung failure.

In the post-death analysis of the case, which included a review of all the tests from the time Marie was four months old, as well as the viewing of selective autopsy tissue, Carrigan and Knox discovered that HHV-6 actively caused infection during most of the child's illness and continued to infect her until her death. Both lobes of her lungs were infested with the virus, as were the lymph nodes, where large quantities of lymphocytes were infected. Her damaged thymus gland was also densely colonized by HHV-6.

Neither CMV nor P. carinii were present in her lungs at autopsy. While Carrigan and Knox noted the possibility that the presence of both or one of the infections might have, at the time of her last admission to hospital, boosted HHV-6 activity, they had little doubt that HHV-6 was the sole cause of Marie's pneumonia and her sad demise.

Carrigan and Knox proposed that Marie's immature immune system could not combat her original HHV-6 infection, which she likely acquired from her mother at birth. Instead of becoming dormant after initially infecting her, the virus remained active and progressively wiped out her immune system. While they did not have clear-cut evidence that events occurred precisely this way, they felt the scenario closely matched the available laboratory data.

As it happened, Marie's case was also the first time anyone had documented the ability of the A variant of HHV-6 to cause fatal

disease, apparently on its own. Highly specialized lab tests revealed that HHV-6A accounted for 99 percent of the infection in
Marie's lungs, 98 percent in her lymph nodes, and 90 percent
in her thymus. Previously such extensive infection by HHV-6 in
an immune-suppressed individual had been caused mainly by the
virus's B variant.

After investigating Marie's tragedy, Knox began to wonder just
how much damage HHV-6 could cause by itself, and particularly in
the lymph nodes of someone who had been diagnosed with AIDS.
She was determined to find out.

THE LINKS MULTIPLY

By early 1994, Konnie Knox had already fulfilled most of the research requirements for her doctoral thesis. She had amassed a weighty sum of data on the role of HHV-6 in the development of AIDS, and had established the groundwork for a fresh scientific assault on the connection between HHV-6 and HIV. The prevailing wisdom inspired by Bob Gallo—that HHV-6 was a co-factor in AIDS—was turning out to be highly oversimplified.

Knox's examination of autopsy tissue from HIV-infected people who died of AIDS had revealed widespread HHV-6 infection. She was particularly impressed by the amount of the viral infection appearing in the lungs. This was a notable finding because about half of the HIV-infected people with AIDS were dying from respiratory problems, mostly as a consequence of infection.

Following her instincts, Knox decided to focus on macrophages, the large scavenger cells that serve as the lungs' first line of defense against a variety of infections. Her autopsy-tissue study had already shown that macrophages were often depleted in the lungs of HIV-infected AIDS patients, and she now wanted to know how HHV-6 was capable of knocking out those cells. Her tests showed that, besides destroying macrophages, HHV-6 interfered with the normal functioning of the scavenger cells by blocking the release of a type of oxidant, a substance the cells normally generate to attack microbes. Knox noted that HIV was not known to be capable of this specific type of action. She concluded that, at the very least, HHV-6 could contribute to the depletion of macrophages in the lungs. This in turn would weaken the immune system, leaving the body vulnerable to a host of infections that were normally well controlled.

Did HHV-6 help HIV destroy macrophages in the lungs? Not necessarily. HHV-6 apparently had the potential to do a brutally effective job on its own. Perhaps HIV was giving HHV-6 a boost, not the other way around. Or, more provocative yet, Knox wondered, was HIV doing any killing in the body, or was HHV-6 the lone assassin? Clearly, heresy was incubating in the Milwaukee wing of AIDS science.

At this time, Knox and Carrigan were given another medical mystery. Like the others, this one revealed the power of HHV-6 to strike hard. It also made Knox more confident that her doctoral thesis project was on target, steadily accumulating evidence on how the virus contributed to AIDS.

Gabrielle, a 14-month-old infant, came down with fever and a bad cough, among other roseola-like symptoms (without the rash) before she suffered a series of seizures several days later and arrived at the hospital unconscious. An initial examination showed Gabrielle's breathing was quick and uneasy. Chest X rays showed signs of pneumonia. A CT-scan suggested that many areas of her brain had been damaged. She tested positive for HIV, an infection doctors believed had been transmitted to her by her mother, a prostitute who had a history of intravenous drug use. (Gabrielle had been cared for by her aunt.)

The doctors did not hold out much hope for Gabrielle. On her second day in the hospital, her breathing was so weak she needed the assistance of a ventilator. Drug therapy was ineffective. She experienced another round of seizures and died three days later.

Working on Gabrielle's case in the lab with Carrigan and technologist Daniel Harrington, Knox found that HHV-6 appeared to have caused the encephalitis, or brain infection. Throughout the cerebral cortex were cells infected predominantly with the A variant of the virus. It was the first time anyone had documented that HHV-6 caused an invasive tissue disease in an infant who was HIV positive. But perhaps the most startling finding of all was that there were only signs of HHV-6, and not HIV.

Yet in the absence of any evidence of HIV actually causing damage to Gabrielle's body, doctors at the hospital presumed that HIV was responsible for her low T-lymphocyte count, a marker of immune suppression. Knox, however, assessed the situation differently. Because of Gabrielle's young age, it was likely that her HHV-6 infection was primary, not reactivated as a result of a drop in immunity. As tests showed, there were no other viral, fungal, or bacterial infections that could have accounted for Gabrielle's damaged immunity. Knox strongly suspected that HHV-6, being the sole cause of the child's brain infection, was also capable of being the sole cause of her immune problems.

More work in the lab led Knox to further appreciate the role HHV-6 could play in AIDS. She noted that blood problems are common in AIDS, but the AIDS scientific community had been far from clear on whether HIV is actually able to disturb the bone marrow's normal blood-manufacturing processes. Knox now wondered whether HIV was really doing anything. Knox's lab studies demonstrated that HHV-6–infected marrow cells—not the HIV-infected ones—blocked the ability of the marrow to produce mature, differentiated cells.

As Carrigan would later say, the lab at this point was really beginning to crackle with excitement and brainstorming. Knox's inroads and her concerns about conventional AIDS wisdom had him fired up as well. The stakes were growing and the potential dangers of paddling against the current drew ever closer. But the researchers were undaunted. They were guided by one powerful instinct: Follow the science.

After all the years of collaboration, Knox now more fully appreciated Carrigan's encouragement and help. He allowed her more space, and they were more in sync with one another. She also valued his courage. In a profession where people ducked for cover at the sign of the slightest controversy, Carrigan stood defiant. He did not back away from anything he felt was scientifically correct.

The next step in their process of discovery was the lymph nodes, the sites in the body where HIV is reputed to be a destructive force. Lymph nodes are usually found in clusters, mostly around the neck, armpits, and groin. They are part of the extensive lymphatic system of vessels, along which they lie, that drains tissue fluid (lymph) back into the bloodstream. The nodes, which are as tiny as pinheads or as large as small beans, are filters that trap microorganisms. The lymphocytes and macrophages they house can neutralize or destroy them. The development of AIDS has largely been viewed as a progressive destruction of the networks of lymphocytes and fibers known as lymphoid tissue. AIDS scientists, however, have been unable to associate the presence of HIV in the lymph nodes with any damage to tissue.

Knox obtained lymph-node biopsies from 10 people positive for HIV and found that all were actively and predominantly infected with HHV-6A. She also discovered the colonization had mostly occurred early on, as suggested by T-4 lymphocyte counts that were higher than the cut-off point of 200, which qualifies someone for an AIDS diagnosis. One HIV-positive individual's biopsy had even produced a count of 711. HHV-6 was clearly active and reproducing itself before AIDS had even been diagnosed.

In the summer of 1994, Donald Carrigan was proud of the lab's achievements. He felt there was remarkable synergy between his ongoing bone-marrow studies and Knox's investigation of the role of HHV-6 in the development of AIDS. Both sets of research involved studying people with suppressed immune systems. The virus seemed to act similarly in AIDS patients as it did in those undergoing marrow transplants. Some of their findings were appearing in prominent journals, and they were beginning to receive modest recognition for their work from other scientists in the field, particularly from those interested in medical problems associated with transplantation.

Still, no research money was forthcoming from the federal government. The research grant proposals they were submitting were being routinely rejected. While it seemed no one was critical of their work, they heard the same refrain again and again: you're researching a very common virus, and we'd rather give our money to other endeavors. Even in the bone marrow–research arena, there was hesitation to accept findings that so common a virus as HHV-6 could do considerable damage. Others had already done research on herpes viruses such as CMV and EBV that caused problems during organ transplantation. The granting agencies did not think that research on yet another herpes virus merited special consideration.

That was one reason why Carrigan's star at Medical College began to fall. Money can move mountains in academe. Lack of funding becomes a major liability. Still, he could take comfort in the lab's latest research in the *New England Journal of Medicine*.

It was based on work by Carrigan and Knox, with Bill Drobyski, a physician in the bone marrow–transplant program, and David Majewski, a lab technologist. Carrigan had been so enthused by the research findings that he had granted Drobyski first authorship, a move considered by Knox to be overly generous, considering the breakthrough nature of the paper. She would later recall that Carrigan ended up as last author on the paper, and because of the way names are excised in scientific references to articles (usually after the first two or three names are cited), few would realize that Carrigan had spearheaded the work. Carrigan would only partly agree with Knox's assessment, adding that Drobyski had been a valued colleague and that he deserved some kudos.

The publication in the journal centers on Agnes, who at the age of 37 received a bone-marrow transplant from a family member in order to fight off a recurrence of Hodgkin's disease, a progressive malignant enlargement of lymphoid tissue. Fourteen days after the transplant, her body began to reject the marrow, resulting in skin problems, and she was treated with antirejection drugs. Two weeks later, she stabilized. But after another two weeks passed and CMV turned up in her blood, doctors put her on antiviral therapy.

Nine weeks later, when she was no longer on antiviral therapy, Agnes developed a brain infection. She became disoriented and had headaches. Brain scans, however, didn't reveal any damage. Just when it looked as if Agnes would rebound from her ordeal, CMV reappeared and she was back on eight more weeks of antiviral therapy. Then CMV disappeared again.

Two weeks after the antiviral therapy ended, Agnes suffered a dramatic loss in her short-term memory. She again was disoriented, incapable of interacting with people, and withdrawn. It seemed as if something was eating into her brain, even though brain scans found nothing of importance happening to her. The scans were wrong: her neurological condition quickly deteriorated and she soon died.

In studying the brain, the pathologist noticed signs of dead cells in one area, but apparently did not look much further and signed out the brain as normal. But it wasn't normal. Carrigan and Knox examined some of the tissue samples prepared on slides and discovered massive destruction of the sheaths of nerve fibers in the brain's white matter (the inner regions rich in nerve fibers), particularly in the frontal lobe of the cerebral cortex. In areas of myelin destruction, axons, the nerve cell extensions that conduct impulses away from the body of the neuron, had also degenerated.

The tests that Carrigan and Knox conducted showed massive HHV-6B infection in this region of the brain, particularly in the large, star-shaped cells known as astrocytes. In white matter that appeared normal, there was no sign of the virus. Further investigation of the autopsy tissue revealed a second area of the brain that had been attacked by HHV-6. Killed cells and dense HHV-6B infection were evident in the gray matter (the outer layer of brain cells) of the hippocampus gyrus, an area important to memory.

From the study of Agnes's brain tissue, it was clear that HHV-6 could infect and destroy the adult central nervous system. Tests for signs of other microbes, including CMV, herpes simplex types 1 and 2, varicella-zoster and, of course, HIV, were negative. Carrigan and Knox had uncovered yet another way HHV-6 could kill. While they could not prove it, they suspected that the infection of Agnes's brain was induced by HHV-6. From that point on, the virus may have progressively destroyed her brain.

But this type of destruction was occurring not only in bone-marrow patients, as the graduate-student half of the Carrigan lab was already demonstrating.

Knox knew she was about to take a big step in her research. It was common for AIDS patients to develop brain damage, particularly the wide range of damage to the sheaths covering nerve fibers. When damage was extensive, it was referred to as AIDS leukoencephalopathy. Autopsy studies have shown that roughly 20 percent of AIDS patients have this condition at the time of death.

Knox was also well aware that such complications are often attributed to HIV, even though the direct role of the virus in causing damage to the central nervous system had never been firmly established. Nor, for that matter, has any indirect role been proven, although theories have circulated about how chemicals emitted by HIV itself or its proteins damage brain cells.

When Knox studied the brains of six people who died of AIDS and found extensive damage in four to their nerve fiber sheaths, she also detected active HHV-6 infection. The infected cells were only in areas where the damage had occurred and never in healthy tissue. The damaged tissue tested negative for signs of HIV, CMV, and other microbes. Again, there was only HHV-6.

Knox marveled at how similar the damage in Agnes's brain was to what she had discovered in studies of people who had died of AIDS. Because Agnes's brain problems were not caused by HIV, Knox reasoned, the brains of AIDS patients were not likely to suffer from HIV either. At this point in the Carrigan lab, she and Carrigan were wondering if HIV was even necessary for AIDS to occur.

*   *   *

In 1982, before Luc Montagnier and Robert Gallo laid claim to HIV, there were numerous scientific discussions about whether CMV was the cause of AIDS.

Joseph Sonnabend, the New York doctor who was one of the first to care for AIDS patients, placed CMV high on the list of key suspects for his multiple-factor theory of how AIDS developed. He had studied many gay men heavily infected by CMV. Donald Francis, a researcher at the Centers for Disease Control in Atlanta, also advanced CMV as a possible cause of AIDS, based on evidence that the virus infected the brains of AIDS patients. Among AIDS researchers at the time, CMV was the most frequent infection known. Before long, CMV gave way to the HIV hypothesis, and then became known only as an infection that occasionally reactivated in the body when immunity was weakened. This suggests why CMV was so often cited as a potentially harmful factor in transplantation.

Fast-forward to the mid-1990s: Carrigan and Knox had so far shown that CMV, while causing trouble in marrow transplants, was not as important in many patients as HHV-6 was. Knox had shown that in the tissue of people who had died of AIDS, infection by HHV-6 was far more prevalent than by CMV, although CMV would pop up time and again and then disappear after antiviral treatment.

Scientists such as Sonnabend, Francis, and the many others who proposed CMV early on as a possible cause of AIDS did not have the benefit of knowing that a similar, but in many ways a more immune-destructive, herpes virus would soon be unearthed by none other than Gallo and his NCI team. What they thought was caused by CMV might at least sometimes, if not often, have been caused by HHV-6.

Research on the brains of AIDS patients produced another startling turn. The discovery was accidental, as is often the case in science.

The focus of all the fuss in the Carrigan lab was the well-preserved brain tissue from Helen, a 27-year-old patient who had died more than 20 years earlier. Her medical records showed that she had been diagnosed with multiple sclerosis, a neurological disease affecting at least 300,000 Americans, women twice as often as men. MS most often wears away at myelin, the sheaths that protect the nerves in the brain and spinal cord, leaving lesions. While left intact, the naked axons, the cylindrical extensions of nerves, become incapable of sending the types of messages required to properly control movements, speech, and a wide range of bodily functions. Symptoms, such as numbness or tingling, weakness, and unsteadiness, often appear abruptly. Usually they go into remission, only to reappear. In time, the physical signs of MS may be accompanied by cognitive troubles, including impaired attention, short-term memory, and thought disorganization. Patients typically endure varying cycles of attacks and remissions; about half will develop some form of progressive disease, some ending up in wheelchairs. While drugs such as interferon beta may cut down on the severity and numbers of attacks, and steroids may cut short some episodes and inflammation, no treatments are considered broadly effective enough to predictably reassure patients that progression of the disease can be halted.

Helen's acute illness had been uncharacteristically rapid and constant. It erupted with weakness in her arms and legs and the inability to walk steadily. Within only a year's time, she was admitted to the hospital several times with such symptoms as partial paralysis, hearing and speech loss, difficulty in swallowing, and facial nerve paralysis. A scan revealed multiple MS-type lesions in her brain's white matter. She also suffered a seizure in the hospital and became incontinent. After finally being moved to a nursing home, Helen lost more of her bodily functions to the disease, including her corneal and gag reflexes. She became comatose and died.

Knox and Carrigan had included Helen's brain tissue in the AIDS study to serve as a control, along with brain tissue from other individuals who had been diagnosed with a neurological disease. They believed those controls would be free of HHV-6 infection. They presumed correctly, except in Helen's case.

Checking their tissue slides in the lab, Knox and Carrigan were dumbfounded. Knox would later refer to her first reaction to the slides as "a scary moment." They found enormous amounts of HHV-6 in both Helen's brain and spinal cord tissue. The infection had been active at the time of her death. Everywhere that myelin had been attacked, they found HHV-6–infected cells within or near the area. In regions where myelin had not been attacked, there was no sign of infected cells.

What was HHV-6 doing in an MS patient? Since it was only found in abnormal brain areas, could it possibly be the cause of MS? While they were certainly not going to jump to any such conclusion, the finding matched what they had discovered in the brains of people with AIDS and transplant patients: The virus appeared to be feasting on myelin. But MS patients didn't have the powerful immunity defects that AIDS patients and bone marrow–transplant recipients did.

The usual explanation for the occurrence of MS is that the body's own immune system launches an inflammatory attack against myelin, namely that lymphocytes behave as though myelin is foreign to the body. Thus, MS has been referred to as an "auto-immune" disease. It is also conventional wisdom that genetics play an important role in determining who is more vulnerable. If a family member has MS, first-degree relatives would have a small additional risk of getting the disease, a jump from a fraction of one percent to a chance roughly of one to three percent.

It has also long been assumed that environmental factors played a triggering role in MS. A wide array of possible toxic substances have been considered, such as lead, pesticides, diesel fumes, and tap water chemicals. But over many years, viruses have been among the chief suspects, including a retrovirus named HTLV-1, measles virus, rubella, and even the canine distemper virus. Not one of these has ever been shown to be active in destroyed neurological tissue in MS patients.

Knox and Carrigan were staring at evidence of such an association. They thought the disease process, in simple terms, might work this way: HHV-6, which is generally attracted to certain nerve cells, attacks the myelin and triggers the immune system to respond to the attack, thus causing inflammation. Unless the virus calms down and goes back to sleep for good, it will continue to periodically, if not chronically, trigger an immune response and the accompanying inflammation. More and more of the brain tissue around this inflammation will get killed and replaced by scar tissue. Over time, the brain tissue will accumulate deficits, culminating in more severe disease.

This was, of course, only theory based on a dazzling but preliminary discovery. Much more research would be required before the link between HHV-6 and MS could be firmly established. In any case, Knox and Carrigan were not about to follow their lead on MS. Their laboratory was funded by some internal college funds only to study AIDS and bone-marrow transplants. There was absolutely no money to study MS, even though they had made a potentially remarkable advance in neurological science. Science can be a miserable discipline, particularly if you are operating a lab at rock bottom. They would have to let the new and explosive data drop. It would take a full year before they could return to MS.

SCENE OF THE CRIME

As far as David Ho was concerned, the question of whether or not HIV caused AIDS was resolved once and for all. In January 1995, he and his colleagues at the Aaron Diamond AIDS Research Center in New York City had made sure of that. Anyone still dense enough to clutter the AIDS science field with fanciful tales of how HIV did not trigger AIDS or of how co-factors were at play could no longer cling to even a thread of credibility.

Preaching from the director's pulpit of one of the best-equipped AIDS laboratories in the United States, Ho had the confidence of someone in his esteemed position. The research center on the seventh floor of New York City's health department building was a luxurious facility where even the laboratory surfaces were marbled. It was created with philanthropic dollars and had gradually maneuvered its way to the forefront of "AIDS hope," the quixotic promise of a breakthrough treatment, and maybe even a cure, for the dreaded syndrome of illnesses. It certainly did not hurt Ho's credibility that he was a fresh, rising star in the AIDS establishment. The Taiwan-born Ho looked more like a young graduate student than a real professional, but to the old guard it was time for fresh troops to replace the tired soldiers fighting valiantly to prove how HIV actually caused damage to the immune system.

In a paper published in the journal *Nature,* Ho and his team in New York (backed by further research by a group from the University of Alabama at Birmingham) made a simple but dramatic claim: HIV was never inactive. From the time of infection, the scientists claimed, HIV reproduced as many as a billion times each day. These viral particles killed the 100 million to one billion T-4 cells produced by the body's immune system each day. The biological seesaw could rage for years before the virus overwhelmed the T-4 cells and immune system. This was the point at which AIDS was diagnosed and when the body began to be overrun by a host of normally harmless infections.

The other news that struck like a thunderbolt was the authors' claim that a combination of powerful experimental antiviral drugs was apparently able to temporarily block HIV from killing T-4 cells, allowing them to replenish and restore their counts. A potential treatment, and possibly the eradication of HIV, might be just around the corner.

Predictably, Ho's theory sent some AIDS researchers into paroxysms of delight. They were not bothered by the fact that the theory was based entirely on a complex mathematical model (in other words, an inference) of how the immune system eventually failed. Neither were they bothered by the scant amount of "therapeutic" data or by the lack of knowledge of longer-term treatment's efficacy. What mattered was that the AIDS science community was finally given an "active" virus to work with and to treat; previously HIV had been portrayed as being latent (inactive), as sitting in the body harmlessly until some event occurred to awaken it.

Some AIDS researchers did not accept Ho's theory, including those who had screened numerous AIDS autopsies. Where was physical evidence that HIV killed immune cells? they wondered. It was one thing to mathematically model a killing spree; it was quite another to examine a crime scene in the flesh with real HIV.

There was no evidence, only theory for the way that HIV kills. The virus triggered what amounted to a complex molecular process that resulted in the death of T-4s. The killing was so quick in the lymph nodes that very few infected cells could escape into the bloodstream. This would explain why blood samples typically showed little sign of T-4 cell infection.

But HIV particles that had not caused cell infection jetted out of the lymph nodes into the bloodstream. The number of these particles when counted by a PCR (polymerase chain reaction) test represented the "viral load." Some AIDS dissidents, including Duesberg, were appalled by the claims that PCR had revealed signs of a huge hidden store of HIV in the blood. First of all, PCR was used to identify HIV RNA (a genetic molecule) as a marker for HIV itself. Second, by running the blood through PCR, whole RNA produced by HIV could not be distinguished from defective bits of HIV and HIV neutralized by antibodies. In other words, the massive amounts of RNA supposedly pointing to HIV circulating in the blood were highly suspect. Was Ho staring at a "viral mirage"?

Even HIV proponents such as Robert Gallo were annoyed by the audacity of Ho claiming credit for a breakthrough. Weren't their findings essentially based on a theory that Gallo, along with others, had proposed early in the AIDS epidemic, namely that the virus overwhelmed T-4 cells? Admittedly, it was a theory Peter Duesberg had forced them all to reconsider, which is when they began fashioning theories of indirect HIV cell-killing methods. Ho had done a modest modification job on the prevailing wisdom. Later, Gallo would say, "Just about everyone knew right from the start [his theory] was absolutely wrong."

Ho had not been the first, however, to find covert signs of HIV in the body. Researchers, including Anthony Fauci, head of the National Institute of Allergy and Infectious Diseases, had previously claimed that massive HIV infection in the lymph nodes of AIDS patients was eluding detection. These findings were also controversial. Some critics pointed out that upon close examination, the numbers of infected cells, compared to those uninfected, in patients, were mostly insignificant. Such a lack of virulence might not have surprised the laboratory scientist working with HIV, who would have been acutely aware of how difficult it was to prime infected cells to generate the virus.

The lack of evidence for powerful infection in the body, and especially for active infection (which destroys tissue) in the lymph nodes, did not appear to concern David Ho. He exuded great confidence in the new theory, convinced that the antivirals had reduced a viral load almost magically, allowing T-4s to rebound. Despite the controversy dogging the new theory, Ho would soon emerge as the undisputed superstar of AIDS science.

Science works in predictable ways, thought Konnie Knox. Credentials, powerful institutions, and journals and networks of like-minded colleagues all contributed to the construction of scientific truths. It was an incestuous dynamic. Fail to respect it and prepare to suffer the consequences professionally. You fail to get the nod from the right person for the right career move. You are not invited to deliver talks. Be daring yet truthful in interpreting a scientific finding even if it means stepping on the toes of fellow scientists, and you are asking for rejection. Science is not a democracy, Knox was learning. Science often punishes people for pursuing the truth.

For months Knox and Carrigan had been very deliberate about how they wrote up their HHV-6–related AIDS papers for publication. On the one hand, they were aggressively advancing the theory of HHV-6 as a co-factor. The title of Knox's 210-page doctoral dissertation was "Human Herpesvirus Six (HHV-6): Evidence for Its Role as a Cofactor in the Pathogenesis of AIDS." On the other, they played down the role the herpes virus played in the development of AIDS, although they knew from both their bone-marrow and AIDS research that HHV-6 appeared to have the power on its own to damage the immune system. On the contrary, when they observed HIV in the test tube, it did little, especially when compared to the powerful killing power of HHV-6. There continued to be a lack of evidence showing HIV killing cells in the lymph nodes, a feature of HIV that was widely claimed to be the hallmark of AIDS.

They also had new findings that seemed to directly contradict David Ho's theory. They had compelling evidence that HHV-6 was destroying cells where it was felt that HIV was the viral culprit: in the lymph nodes. "Great timing," Carrigan exclaimed ruefully. "Just when everyone was getting excited about HIV hiding out in the lymph nodes and circulating in the blood."

The latest results were straightforward yet provocative: 16 lymph-node biopsies from HIV-positive patients all contained cells actively infected with HHV-6A. Twelve of 16 patients who had been diagnosed with progressive disease had more dense infection than the four patients who had been diagnosed as having a stable condition. Knox and Carrigan also found more dense infection in areas where the lymph nodes were losing lymphocytes than in areas free of destructive change or where normal tissue in the nodes was already being replaced by the formation of scar tissue. HHV-6 was the apparent cause of the destruction of lymphoid tissue that occurred in these HIV-positive people.

HHV-6 was not only at the scene of the crime, but it appeared to have committed the crime as well. While the evidence was not conclusive, it was closer than Knox and Carrigan had ever come in their detective work. In contrast, there were no convincing studies demonstrating that HIV could cause similar pathology. Studying the findings, Knox and Carrigan looked at one another and wondered if they'd found a smoking gun.

NOVEMBER SONG

**Medical College of Wisconsin, Milwaukee
November 1995**

It had been quite a year for Donald Carrigan, a roller-coaster 11 months of triumphs and an equal number of disappointments. He was experienced enough as a scientist to accept both the highs and the lows, the days when the hairs on his arm seemed to stand on end with excitement followed by days when he wondered why he bothered with it all.

Research in the lab had been thriving, thanks in no small measure to Konnie Knox and her investigations into AIDS. She had pushed the envelope, creating an adventure for them both. At times Carrigan had been unnerved, feeling they needed to be absolutely right about the profile they were creating for HHV-6. Knox did not share such a fear. She had no problem admitting to a mistake and then getting on with the work. Being a mother to five children likely made her more flexible and forgiving. Science was Carrigan's entire life. It was just one part of Knox's.

Their working relationship had continued to be tense, but productively so. Knox had lip, and Carrigan was no wallflower. The combination had made for legendary blow-ups over the tiniest of points, but out of it had come bushels of quality research, a dozen papers published that year alone in high-profile journals. Their transplant research had been methodical and precise, clearly exposing HHV-6's potential to be a monster. Now they had more knowledge of what it could do, they thought perhaps some of the antiviral treatments being tested at other hospitals could save lives. But they still needed to get more transplant doctors to pay attention to their findings. The doctors needed to test for HHV-6 and attack it quickly before it could invade and suppress the marrow. With transplants being used with greater frequency for blood disorders, cancers, AIDS, and marrow failures, the stakes were getting much higher.

The problem was that doctors could not just test for HHV-6, treat for it, and send the patient home with little or no follow-up. Look what had happened to Fred, their first case: He recovered from pneumonia, returned home, and just when it appeared that he was making a strong recovery, the virus struck again, this time in the marrow. HHV-6 probably was never knocked out completely when he was being treated in hospital. Instead it likely persisted at a low level before flaring up when his defenses were weakened. It was clear that treating chronic HHV-6 infection with antivirals would not be a one-shot deal.

Knox and Carrigan's findings had become increasingly complex. Now it appeared that variant A was more virulent in suppressing bone marrow than the B variant. In one case, a woman infected with both had turned up with all her bone-marrow blood-cell manufacturing nearly destroyed almost two years after her marrow transplant. Perhaps the two variants worked more efficiently together than apart, Knox and Carrigan thought. Doctors could not stop being vigilant for HHV-6 reactivation a few months after surgery just because infection was known usually to occur much sooner.

By this point Knox and Carrigan were frustrated by how slowly their ideas were working their way into the medical world, by how little encouragement they were receiving, even from their own department and college. They had had little time to promote their ideas, being preoccupied by all the research that still needed to be done. They knew the virus was common and was difficult to sift out as a destructive entity. They knew that in the case of people who were HIV-positive, controlled long-term studies would be required to narrow down when HHV-6 began to play a role in damaging the immune system and how it contributed to the progression of AIDS. Yes, it would be terrific to have clinical trials to see whether antiviral treatment against HHV-6 in AIDS patients made a difference. They knew all this, but they could do only so much themselves. And there was still the matter of funding: no one was getting much money to do research on HHV-6. Their find on multiple sclerosis could be monumental, but there was no money to continue on that track.

Carrigan realized that a major problem was not about to go away: HHV-6 science was often considered soft because tests used by researchers to detect the virus varied so widely. There were no common standards. One unfortunate development was the indiscriminate use of PCR, fast becoming an ill-advised shortcut. Research by a team from the University of Washington and the Fred Hutchinson Cancer Research Center, both in Seattle, was a case in point. The Seattle researchers examined lung biopsies from patients with pneumonia after marrow transplants and found a strong association between HHV-6 and pneumonia. They had published their results in the *New England Journal of Medicine* in 1993. Several scientists who had read the report wrote letters to the journal cautioning that any suggestion that a causal relationship between HHV-6 and any disease, such as pneumonia, was premature. The Seattle team responded by voicing its gratitude to the letter writers, stating that the biopsy research had never concluded that HHV-6 had actually caused the pneumonia. The researchers had only associated the virus with pneumonia. Of course, Carrigan and Knox believed they had demonstrated that HHV-6 very likely was the cause in some immune-suppressed patients of the same type of pneumonia. They had shown that the more dense the infected cells were, the more tissue damage could be observed. It might not have been final proof, but it was close enough for them to be quite confident.

The experience with the Seattle team showed clearly how HHV-6 researchers too often used inappropriate technology to look for the virus, in the process casting a shadow on all HHV-6 research. The Seattle researchers had used a type of PCR to probe the lymph nodes, a technology with clear limitations that could confuse the genetic sequences of viruses with those produced by damaged cells. The test could also miss detection of low-level active infections, confusing them with inactive ones. Yet even low-level active infections could trigger disease, including inflammation, immune reactions, and bone-marrow suppression. Carrigan felt the scientists should have used one of several rigorous techniques to isolate active virus in the lymph nodes. Such techniques, which allow the closest look at what the virus was doing, show a positive result only when the infection is active in the blood or tissues. This is the gold standard in virology, a standard that clearly was not being used often enough. It was time-consuming, expensive, and good lab experience was necessary, but so what? Carrigan and Knox, always on a tight lab budget, had managed to use isolation techniques.

All of these science-related concerns, though, were becoming overshadowed by a more alarming development. The lab where they had done so much work would soon be taken from them.

This had already happened to Knox three months earlier, in August. The problem had been building for many months. There was no budget and office space allotted to her after she had completed her doctoral degree. Medical College bureaucrats refused to budge on the issue: Knox had to go. Here was someone who had been given an award by the college for best doctoral dissertation, who had been published in major science journals. "Anyone with even limited brain power would have tried to keep her and treat her well," Carrigan said, his face reddening.

Knox had desperately taken a lab job nearby at St. Luke's Medical Center doing genetic research. They were already restricting her, not letting her work on HHV-6. Because she and Carrigan still had papers to write, they began to meet daily in the hospital coffee shop and work together to complete their projects. Their lunch table was usually overflowing with books, lab data, science journals, and grant applications. It was an offbeat way to do science, but what choice did they have?

"I was worried about Don. He looked tired and troubled. He

would show up each day at the coffee shop with a package of material—lab data and drafts of scientific papers—for me to review.
Then we would make plans to continue our research together,
both knowing this might become more and more difficult."

There was another reason for concern: Carrigan had also been
given the boot at Medical College. He finally had made it impossi-
ble for the bureaucrats to keep him. His contract was not renewed,
and he had one school year left in the lab. "Some of his hassles
were on my behalf, but others were just Don being Don."

For the next year, his department would pretend he did not
even exist. They did not appear to care that he had been a highly
productive lab scientist and director. He had been laid low by personality and politics.

Carrigan had never faced such a situation before. Jobs would
not come easy. As an accomplished scientist, he would be expected
to come to an institution with buckets of scientific grant money,
particularly from the National Institutes of Health. But that was
not going to happen. The one option Carrigan could think of was
to accept a job in the pharmaceutical industry, hardly his idea of a
good time.

Knox wondered with growing concern about whether Carrigan
would stay in Milwaukee. She feared their hard work on HHV-6
would soon stop for good.

Yet as that year drew to a close, Carrigan decided that he would
stick out his final year at Medical College and continue to work
with Knox on HHV-6. For now, it meant meeting Knox day after
day in the St. Luke's coffee shop.

He knew his decision was a huge gamble. If they couldn't find a
way to do research at a proper lab, they would be at a huge disad-
vantage in the effort to impress anyone with any further medical
detective work. Science runs on reputation. The names Harvard or
Yale have currency. Even Medical College merits an ear or two.
But not Coffee Shop.

Carrigan and Knox remained focused on HHV-6, thinking up
research grants that they might write in the hope of one day ending their exile and returning to laboratory detective work. They
therefore weren't paying much attention to some scientific devel-

opments that potentially could have a bearing on their HHV-6 adventure. These included provocative challenges that HIV was not a real virus and therefore not the cause of AIDS. Emerging were intriguing theories that controversial and difficult-to-diagnose illnesses, including multiple sclerosis and chronic fatigue syndrome, were part of a constellation of virally induced central nervous system disorders. Also being raised were concerns that certain vaccines might harbor monkey viruses, including herpes viruses, that could potentially either recombine with other genetic material to pose grave threats to human health or directly provoke the immune system into a dangerous tailspin. Those were all ideas that were beginning to receive a broader public airing, and were already seen by some advocates as planting the seeds for a badly needed total reevaluation of how complex and chronic diseases emerge.

In this context, Carrigan and Knox were actually middle-of-the-road in their scientific thinking and objectives. At one extreme were the established ideas, say, of AIDS and MS, and at the other extreme were the bold new theories clamoring for recognition.

Carrigan and Knox had been contributing important pieces of HHV-6 science to a complex scientific jigsaw puzzle that could go a long way to change how we think about chronic disease and how to medically intervene. Yet without a lab, how could they continue?

There would be a prolonged silence from the productive team. The new viral theories would continue to evolve. And by the time Carrigan and Knox were back on their feet, they would find that others had been investigating similar lines of inquiry, lines that were all starting to converge.

A SALVO FROM
DOWN UNDER

Perth is a city of one million people located on the southwest coast of Australia, 7,000 miles from Milwaukee. In December 1995 a five-member research group at the Royal Perth Hospital, led by medical biophysicist Eleni Papadopulos-Eleopulos, made the charge that AIDS scientists had made a colossal error in declaring HIV as the cause of AIDS. Theirs was not more of the same type of criticism that had been leveled at HIV science. Unlike California maverick Peter Duesberg who claimed HIV did not cause AIDS, the Perth Group had instead raised the stakes—by questioning the very existence of HIV. They claimed the virus had never been properly identified and that all of HIV science stood on a foundation of sand. The team's most recent appraisal of HIV published in the summer of 1995 in the journal *Genetica* was by far the most fastidious academic attack to date on HIV theory.

The Perth Group's provocation attracted the attention of *Continuum*, a London-based science magazine critical of HIV theory. The magazine decided to offer an award of 1,000 British pounds to anyone who could cite one scientific paper that provided proof that a virus called HIV had been extracted from the body in a manner that followed certain established rules for identifying a retrovirus. The magazine hoped that putting up some money for an award might draw out some AIDS scientists and help stimulate a debate about HIV. While some critics of HIV applauded the magazine's offer, they could not deny that the scheme seemed like a sideshow come-on. Its offering highlighted how much of a fortress had been built around the HIV theory and its defenders disdained any academically sanctioned public forum for competing views of how AIDS developed.

It is interesting to note that, painstakingly focused on HIV, the Perth Group had not cited Carrigan and Knox among the 167 scientific references in their report in *Genetica*. Hard pressed to keep up with research in their own highly specialized domains, scientists often remain ignorant of data related to their work until someone shows them the new material. Even after this information gap is breached, new ideas still may not have much immediate impact. Like most people, scientists generally do not change or broaden theories in which they have invested so much effort. Had Carrigan and Knox and the Australians somehow managed to share their respective theories and data, they might have realized that each was adding to, and reinforcing, the other's evolving perspective on HIV and AIDS.

In any case, back in 1983, Eleni Papadopulos-Eleopulos had been the first to propose that AIDS was not caused by an exogenous (coming from outside the body) virus. Her suspicions were based on the fact that AIDS cases were distributed within so-called "risk groups," such as homosexuals and hemophiliacs. Some members of these risk groups were exposed to "stressors"—not a new virus—that gradually damaged cells in the body. For instance, many gay men who were heavy users of a variety of street drugs were also taking nitrites to boost their sexual potency. To stem an array of sex-related infections, these same men were consuming great quantities of conventional medicines such as antibiotics that also had immune-suppressing potential. Some also played the passive role in thousands of anal sex encounters with a wide variety of partners. As a result, the multitude of such toxic "hits," including those from semen, could trigger the release of oxidizing, or cell-damaging, chemicals known as free radicals.

The same cell-damaging process also held true for hemophiliacs, Papadopulos-Eleopulos believed, because in the blood-clotting product they received, known as factor 8, they were bombarded with immune-altering foreign blood cells. Street-drug users, many suffering the immune-suppressing effects of malnutrition, were further susceptible to cell damage as a result of excessive injection and inhalation of powerful narcotics. In Africa, impoverished people had to fight off rampant disease, which also caused cellular damage leading to immune suppression. In fact, the scientific literature offered abundant evidence that these and other types of oxidative attacks on cells could lower the number of vital T-4 lymphocytes. There was no need, the Australian scientist believed, to call upon a new virus to achieve this result.

When HIV had been introduced by Montagnier and Gallo as the likely cause of AIDS, Papadopulos-Eleopulos begged to differ. Retroviruses were not known to kill cells; therefore, how could they kill T-4 lymphocytes? There was no evidence showing that HIV killed cells.

As the Perth Group later claimed, neither Montagnier nor Gallo had followed some fundamental rules in molecular biology to adequately extract what they claimed was a retrovirus from human cells. Isolating a virus, they argued, requires separating it from everything else biological that goes on in cells. One well-established way to achieve this is to place the biological specimen in a centrifuge that measures density, since various densities are associated with certain viruses. The specimen is spun until particles of the virus band at a particular level. Once this banding occurs, particles can then be systematically photographed and studied with an electron microscope and probed to determine their exact genetic makeup and to determine whether they are infectious. In its paper in *Genetica,* the Perth Group charged that not one HIV scientist—including Montagnier and Gallo—had ever detected pure HIV by using what they believed was the "gold standard" of isolating a retrovirus.

The HIV pioneers had felt confident with their discovery because they had detected the enzyme reverse transcriptase, which had been first proposed in 1970 as a marker for retroviruses, and largely on that basis believed they had isolated HIV. But the Perth group thought it was wrong to presume that the enzyme was associated only with retroviruses. Retrovirologists had already learned that reverse transcriptase occurs in all living things. So, according to the Australians, the enzyme should not be used as a marker solely for a retrovirus.

What, then, could HIV possibly be? The Perth Group posited that the biological material characterized as HIV might very well have originated in human cells, from any one of the hundreds or thousands of ancient genetic sequences lying dormant in human DNA that are passed from one generation to the next. Such genetic material might awaken and behave like a life form (a retrovirus) when cells are damaged: potentially reproducing itself and making genetic products, including proteins. There is evidence which shows that this process is greatly accelerated once cells come under heavy attack from a variety of toxic substances. In other words, diseased cells can give rise to so-called retroviruses. Perhaps AIDS occurs first as cells become damaged and only then does the endogenous retroviral material emerge. Once it does, its proteins are seen as foreign by the immune system and they are attacked, thus producing specific antibodies.

Given these possibilities, the Perth Group concluded, it was absolutely essential to ensure that HIV, said to be an exogenous retrovirus, was not being confused with internally generated retroviruses.

The Perth Group also said that the way HIV was grown in the laboratory did not ensure that a pure virus emerged. AIDS researchers had developed a culture—a biochemical soup—from a recipe of long-living leukemia cells that served as a base for growing the "virus." It was supposedly contained in extracts of human cells that were released into the soup. Only HIV proved to be a very difficult virus to grow. Because it needed a powerful biochemical boost, researchers added plant extracts and other chemicals to the soup to prime the cells to begin producing copies of itself. In the end, even after the drastic manipulation of the soup, all the researchers could typically detect was reverse transcriptase, not a virus.

The Perth Group contended that no separate, "outside" virus emerged from that soup. The variable stretches of genetic material that HIV scientists occasionally extracted and regarded as evidence of HIV's viral code were far more likely the by-products of activated biological material that was part of every human cell. As well, the Australians pointed out that the soup was exactly the type of toxic environment that could generate new genetic products, combining the human material with the soup's agents. The plant extracts and chemicals were certainly capable of triggering damage to cells. Those cells, in turn, could trigger the emergence of new genetic materials, mistakenly attributed to a so-called virus from outside the body named HIV.

It is easy to see why mainstream HIV researchers might hesitate to explore in any detail the theory proposed by the Perth Group. The idea that HIV is really genetic material arising out of cells—and possibly harmless material at that—seemed too outlandish to those who had spent years determined to solve the mystery of how HIV destroys the immune system. Should the Perth Group prevail, it would mean that thousands of scientists worldwide had wasted their time. There had been powerful political pressure to find the cause of the syndrome, and soon after, the funding for HIV research became so plentiful. Under the right political and economic conditions and the pressures of peer persuasion, it is not inconceivable that science can build huge edifices on the barest of scientific findings. And once the edifice is built, it is extremely difficult to dismantle.

Over time, media reports of one aspect or another of the established view strongly reinforce it in the minds of the public. Most people would by now have a difficult time considering AIDS to be non-infectious, as the Perth Group's theory contends. When we think of AIDS, it's hard not to think in terms of a transmissible agent—as a killer virus that can infect anyone who, for example, uses unclean needles to shoot up drugs or doesn't practice safe sex. When we think of AIDS, we think of being either positive or negative for HIV. This medical concept has become deeply ingrained in our culture.

It hasn't helped the cause of the Perth Group that Peter Duesberg disagrees with their theory. He believes, for example, that since certain genetic sequences have been found in the culture "soup," this represents an isolation of the virus. He also advances the view held by mainstream scientists that people who show signs of HIV DNA in their bodies also make antibodies to HIV. And those who lack HIV DNA do not produce such antibodies.

The Perth Group has responded to his critique by claiming that the genetic sequences in the culture soup are all unlike each other, that there is so much genetic variation among these "isolates" (as much as 40 percent) that it raises serious questions about whether they can be described as representing a unique virus. The Perth Group adds that the antibodies produced in the HIV test may be reacting to endogenous genetic material that is activated when people become ill, thus explaining the difference between those who turn up positive and negative. Those who are not ill are not likely to have damaged cells and therefore no ancient genetic materials become activated in those cells.

As for mainstream HIV researchers, some have dismissed out of hand the Australian theory. To their way of thinking, once you can grow a virus and reveal some of its genetic sequences, you clearly have a virus. It is therefore inevitable that the highly complex issue of whether HIV has been truly isolated and whether it is a real virus or not will continue to be controversial for some time.

One intriguing outgrowth of the Perth Group's theory is that it might help explain the importance of HHV-6 in AIDS. As Carrigan and Knox had discovered, when cells become damaged, HHV-6, dormant in the body, is more likely to awaken. Similarly, HHV-6, upon being transmitted from one body, might enter another, stressed-out body and cause havoc there.

If, in fact, HIV does turn out to be endogenous and possibly harmless, then it might mean that anyone who is positive for HIV, and therefore showing signs of cell damage, might be vulnerable to activation of HHV-6. This scenario would help to explain why people with AIDS who have experienced such sustained insults, such as the long-term effects of street drugs or antibiotics, usually are positive for HIV, but show no signs of damage from that virus.

Their bodies, as revealed by Carrigan and Knox, are being damaged by HHV-6.

This remains theoretical, however. What cannot be disputed about the Perth Group's paper is that it was a call to widen the field of investigation into how viruses operate inside the human body. Another scientist, from California this time, was launching a simultaneous attack, one that would not only cast doubt on the HIV establishment, but the world of vaccines as well.

INOCULATION OR CONTAMINATION?

Microbiologist Howard Urnovitz had a habit of working late in his office at the biotech firm he had founded in 1988. From all that hard work had come a host of recent accomplishments, such as his co-authorship set for early in the new year in *Clinical Microbiology Reviews* of an exhaustive and esoteric scientific paper on how endogenous retroviruses might be involved in disease. He viewed his contribution on the subject of those mysterious genetic fragments that have, over the millennia, interwoven themselves into the genetic material of human cells as representing his most impressive scholarship to date.

There are two prominent aspects to Urnovitz's highly energetic personality: a studious, workaholic side that any slacker would find demoralizing, and a maverick tilt that brazenly tested the scientific waters in search of "truth," an elusive commodity he believed was sometimes obscured by gross incompetence or stonewalling. Urnovitz didn't bother to hide his distaste for scientists who were resistant to public review of their cherished principles. Science advances by being challenged. That is, at least in theory, its very essence. He'd gladly take up the issue with any scientist who behaved otherwise, especially some of the top dogs in AIDS research who, when challenged, had acquired the habit of denouncing everyone who disagreed with HIV conventions as irresponsible.

Yet Urnovitz somehow managed to walk the tightrope of being appreciated by both mainstream scientists and radicals. Perhaps it was his disarming, crackling sense of humor that helped to keep the daggers at bay when he questioned conventional wisdom. His research association with high-profile scientists such as Luc Montagnier afforded him unspoken protection. Also, his primary affiliation with the biotech industry rather than academe also kept him at a remove from a college's bureaucratic demands that sometimes sabotage free exchange of ideas. Even so, Urnovitz was fortunate to retain credibility in the scientific community. He was, after all, challenging well-established HIV theory and raising concerns about the safety of America's most highly honored medical products: vaccines, particularly polio vaccines. In American science in the 1990s, it would have been difficult to choose more hallowed icons to question than HIV and polio vaccines. To include both in a single scientific critique would appear to most scientists to be professionally suicidal, but it was, however, cheeky chutzpah—in other words, pure Urnovitz.

Unlike the Perth Group, which questioned the existence of a virus named HIV, Urnovitz presumed that HIV was real, but he didn't think it was, as then commonly believed, a retrovirus that had somehow jumped from primates to humans in Africa to set the stage for the AIDS epidemic. Retroviruses were not known to kill cells; they instead became part of the genetic makeup of cells. Was science now to believe that a retrovirus transferred from an animal to a human suddenly began killing immune cells, causing AIDS?

According to Urnovitz, the first signs of HIV, discovered by Montagnier's group, was more likely a "chimera," a hybrid of an animal virus and human genetic material. One possibility was that the monkey virus named SIV (Simian Immunodeficiency Virus) had entered humans by way of contaminated polio vaccines, and had combined with sequences of human genes often referred to as endogenous retroviruses. Urnovitz believed that such a recombinant monkey-human virus might then, via a complex and still mysterious biological process, be involved in AIDS. Perhaps this chimera was only helping the real cause of AIDS to devastate the immune system. Or perhaps it appeared only when the body was already being assailed by the real killer of the immune system. In this case, the chimera would be only a biological marker revealing that the body was being damaged.

To Urnovitz, the need to pursue an alternative theory of AIDS, in light of what he held to be an unsatisfactory track record of AIDS science, was not only perfectly reasonable, it was imperative.

To understand how he linked SIV with polio vaccines, a little history of the vaccines would be helpful. With polio epidemics reaching a peak in the United States in the early 1950s, there was a desperate need for a vaccine to prevent the crippling disease. While most people who became infected with the poliomyelitis virus showed only flu-like symptoms, thousands became paralyzed when their nervous systems became infected. In 1952, for example, almost 60,000 Americans became ill, more than 20,000 became paralyzed, and about 3,000 died. The disease struck people from all walks of life. It was unpredictable. Parents were terrified that their children would suddenly become infected. This wasn't only the case in the United States. Polio was widespread throughout the world.

Relief finally arrived with the announcement in April 1955 that Jonas Salk, then at the University of Pittsburgh, had completed successful clinical tests of an injectable vaccine for polio. The vaccine used three strains of poliomyelitis viruses that had been chemically inactivated with formaldehyde in such a way that it still allowed the body's immune system to respond to it and generate protective antibodies. Because it was believed that the Salk vaccine might not provide optimal immunity (because the injected inactivated virus would enter the body via the skin rather than the mouth and digestive tract, as it usually did), work continued on a live, weakened virus vaccine, a type that would not require booster shots and could be administered orally. In 1960, such a vaccine, developed by the National Institutes of Health's Albert Sabin, was given the official government nod over a similar vaccine developed by Hilary Koprowski of the Wistar Institute in Philadelphia. The choice of Sabin's vaccine might have been due to scientific politics rather than any important difference between the two vaccines; various accounts suggest Sabin's closeness to the NIH establishment was the real reason. Before long, his vaccine had replaced Salk's in most countries. In 1997, however, a federal advisory committee on immunizations recommended that both vaccines be used: Salk's to prevent polio from being caused by the live Sabin vaccine and Sabin's to offer the best possible immunization.

In reviewing the available scientific record on polio vaccines, Urnovitz was disturbed by a 1958 study documenting that at least 26 different monkey viruses could contaminate polio vaccines. This was because poliovirus preparations used for vaccines were grown in rhesus and African green monkey kidney cells, which were likely to harbor numerous microbes. The findings included microbial groups which appeared to be monkey counterparts of human viruses such as adenoviruses (causing eye, respiratory, and gastrointestinal system infections), echoviruses (causing, for example, complications in bacterial or viral diseases), and coxsakieviruses (for example, causing hand, foot, and mouth disease). The tests had also detected signs of herpes-like viruses.

Also, polio vaccines given to millions of people from about 1955 to 1963 (possibly 100 million in the United States alone) had been contaminated with SV40, which was said to be a monkey cancer virus. This raised the possibility that SV40 could cause cancers over time in many Americans. This issue would flare up many years later as a major health controversy.

The discovery of SV40 in polio vaccines meant that SIV, discovered in monkeys in 1985 (and found to be related to HIV), might also have eluded detection and entered humans unknowingly to cause AIDS. Urnovitz was intrigued by the research of several individuals which had led them to this controversial conclusion.

The pursuits of Walter Kyle, a Massachusetts attorney, were eye-opening. Kyle began to investigate polio vaccines in the late 1970s after one of his female clients contracted polio from her daughter soon after she had been given the oral Sabin vaccine. Kyle was incensed that individuals might not know that it was possible in rare instances to acquire polio in this manner. In preparing the case for trial, he gained access to numerous documents from Lederle Laboratories, the vaccine's manufacturer. Among them were memos revealing that the company had been having a tough time getting rid of monkey contaminants in its vaccine-production process. Microbes such as foamy viruses, SV40, adenoviruses, and monkey cytomegalovirus were being discovered in the monkey-kidney tissue preparations for the polio vaccine. In scouring the scientific literature, Kyle also learned that tests for cytomegalovirus, a major contaminant in commercial African green monkey tissue, were far from foolproof. He believed the virus might have escaped into some batches of the vaccine. The company denied this.

Kyle later came to believe that SIV, a retrovirus, could have been released in doses of polio vaccines prior to its discovery in 1985. This he suggested in a *Lancet* article in 1992. He had, for example, learned that in 1977 the FDA had been concerned about the possibility that some vaccine might contain retroviruses but ended up releasing the batch. Kyle didn't think the FDA had done sufficient testing to warrant the release. He believed that the vaccine might have been contaminated with SIV and could have been the trigger for AIDS.

While Urnovitz was intrigued by Kyle's thesis about SIV, he nonetheless didn't think that SIV could have evolved so quickly following vaccination to cause AIDS. Instead he felt decades, if not even centuries, would be required to make an effective leap from monkeys to humans. He had the same reaction in 1994 when the journal *Medical Hypothesis* published a thesis by Raphael Stricker, a microbiologist at the University of California at San Francisco, and Brian Elswood, a graduate student and AIDS activist. They suggested that experimental polio vaccinations given to 320,000 infants and children in the Belgian Congo between 1957 and 1959 might have given rise to the AIDS epidemic in the region because the vaccine was contaminated. This was the live, weakened vaccine credited to Hilary Korpowski.

While this issue simmered (and would come to a boil again in 1999), Urnovitz believed that it was more likely that SIV and human genetic material had combined to create a biological entity, maybe a virus, that was involved in AIDS. This was something that could happen very quickly.

In any case, Urnovitz's concerns about the polio vaccine went far beyond AIDS. He believed that vaccination in general was a huge area in medicine that required a thorough examination.

Urnovitz had also been working on an innovative study involving Gulf War veterans. About 70,000 soldiers had returned from the war complaining of chronic fatigue–like symptoms (usually referred to as "Gulf War Syndrome"). Most had been required prior to leaving for the Gulf to take as many as 17 different vaccines, including those for polio, cholera, hepatitis B, influenza, anthrax, plague, rabies, tetanus, and yellow fever. They were also given pyridostigmine bromide, an experimental anti-nerve gas.

Urnovitz showed in a blood survey that the soldiers, whether they had been deployed or not, had difficulty building an immune reaction to one version of the live polio vaccine. Deployed soldiers failed to mount a reaction to still another version of the vaccine. In contrast, those noncombatants tested reacted normally. The numerous vaccines the soldiers had taken seemed to have altered their immune systems, potentially making them more vulnerable than usual to environmental toxins in the war zone. Was this assault on immunity the source of at least some of the symptoms that were disabling these returning soldiers? Urnovitz suspected that this was the case and was preparing to present his data to a congressional hearing on Gulf War Syndrome scheduled for early in the new year.

Urnovitz's study also raised questions about the safety of taking a polio vaccine simultaneously with so many other vaccines. The federal government guidelines for using live polio vaccine recommended that it not be used whenever other simultaneously used drugs or treatments can weaken the immune system. This could make the person vaccinated more susceptible to toxic agents of one sort or another that could further reduce immune function and cause harm to the central nervous system.

By raising safety questions about vaccines given to the Gulf War soldiers, Urnovitz was addressing an issue far larger than the potential monkey virus contamination of polio vaccines. For example, to what extent were the dozen or more vaccines given to most children by the age of two to fight off diseases such as measles, rubella, mumps, meningitis, tetanus, and hepatitis potentially damaging to their immune systems over the long term? Could these common vaccines be at the root of some chronic neurological diseases? Although immunologists have generally agreed that vaccination may alter the way the immune system functions, the fact was, this major therapeutic thrust of modern medicine remained largely uncharted territory, even at a time when scores of new vaccines were under development. Most vaccines were actually tested only for short-term side effects and not tracked over the long term for more complex reactions.

Urnovitz believes that better understanding of how vaccines might contribute to chronic disease could open up new theoretical and practical paths in medicine. Syndromes such as AIDS and chronic fatigue would likely be viewed very differently. He also believes that vaccines are capable of setting off dangerous latent infections in the body, including HHV-6.

Such mysterious interconnections were bothering other scientists. Another field, chronic fatigue syndrome, was also receiving scrutiny. Was this really "yuppie flu," or was something more sinister, a virus that could evade detection by the immune system, at work?

STEALTH VIRUS

Like AIDS, chronic fatigue syndrome seemed to materialize from thin air. At least that is how Paul Cheney and Daniel Peterson felt when the two doctors in private practice in Incline Village, a Nevada resort town on the northeast shore of Lake Tahoe, were deluged by more than 100 patients who turned up at their office complaining of disabling fatigue, aching muscles, swollen lymph nodes, and flu-like symptoms. Some townfolk, who were angered by the bad-for-business publicity the cluster of medical cases was generating, scoffed at the so-called epidemic. Surely this was some sort of "yuppie flu," they said. Wasn't it interesting that most of the patients were well educated and affluent? Tearing around on burned-out cylinders, no doubt.

But the symptoms their patients exhibited appeared real enough to Cheney and Peterson. They thought the cause might be Epstein-Barr virus, the herpes virus long associated with mononucleosis. Since mono brings on weakness and fatigue, EBV appeared to be a strong candidate. Initial blood tests of patients suggested that Cheney and Peterson were on track, but later government studies also detected elevated levels of the virus in so-called healthy people. So the doctors continued their hunt.

Unexpectedly, several blood samples that Cheney and Peterson sent to a lab in Los Angeles showed signs of a retrovirus infection. It was HTLV-1, the controversial virus which had been linked to T-cell leukemia by Japanese scientists and the Gallo lab at NCI. Other scientists doubted claims for HTLV-1 because the vast majority of people with signs of the virus in their blood appear perfectly healthy. For example, less than one in 100 people exposed to the virus in Japan, where it is quite common, have developed leukemia. While Gallo claimed that the virus would cause leukemia over several decades (just as he claimed HIV would eventually cause AIDS), some of his critics dismissed HTLV-1 as merely a passenger virus that plays no role in disease. In any case, Cheney and Peterson were excited by the Los Angeles laboratory results. They initially thought they might have identified the cause of CFS.

Their viral roller-coaster ride continued when another lab showed no sign of a retroviral infection. Still hoping that HTLV-1 was the culprit, Cheney asked Elaine DeFreitas, an immunologist at the Wistar Institute in Philadelphia, known for its research on the virus, to check out some blood samples. Again, no go. Meanwhile, the term "yuppie flu" was catching on, especially in the media.

Was CFS an organic condition or not? Disease processes with wide variability and lacking stable markers for diagnosis usually become controversial. Cheney and Peterson and many other doctors seeing a steady flow of patients were convinced that they were confronting a complex biological disease, likely one that involved damage to the immune system. Perhaps when immunity was weakened, viruses dormant in human cells awakened and began damaging tissues. Or perhaps a virus triggered the immune system to become hyperactive, causing it to begin attacking itself. The research data usually offered in support of these theories, though, were preliminary, weak, or inconsistent. Other doctors unconvinced of the case for damaged immunity instead looked to stress and battle fatigue as an explanation. In Britain, where cases were also turning up in droves, a team of doctors from London's Charing Cross Hospital even suggested that hyperventilation due to extreme exhaustion and stress accounted for the numerous symptoms. And so it went.

In March 1988, Stephen Strauss, a doctor at the National Institute of Allergy and Infectious Diseases, advanced what would become largely seen by most health care professionals as the federal government's position on chronic fatigue syndrome. Strauss postulated that it was a "psychoneurotic disease." It boiled down to a more sophisticated way of saying "yuppie flu." Strauss's assessment of the condition would stick, and he would become the government's "expert." Federal research funding for CFS would not likely be soaring anytime soon. Sufferers of chronic fatigue-like symptoms were being written off as malingerers by family, friends, employers, and insurance companies.

Paul Cheney left Nevada to set up a medical practice in Charlotte, North Carolina, and by 1988 he had seen enough people with the condition to become more convinced than ever that it was an immune system–related disease. A few of his patients even had illnesses resembling AIDS. Mostly their T-4 lymphocytes were depleted, and some were developing skin problems, including acne and a fungal infection called thrush, which causes painful sores on the tongue. Unlike AIDS, they were not contracting any lethal infections, and their descending T-4 lymphocyte counts eventually stabilized. Still, Cheney was so taken by the immune dysfunction that in May 1989, in testimony before a Senate subcommittee, he suggested that CFS was somehow related to AIDS and urged that its relationship to the AIDS epidemic be investigated.

In June 1990, microbiologist Nancy Klimas and her colleagues at the University of Miami added support to the idea that CFS resulted from immune system abnormalities. They reported in the *Journal of Clinical Microbiology* that all 30 subjects diagnosed with CFS that they had studied were immune-deficient. They highlighted numerous immune abnormalities, including signs that natural killer cells were functioning at low ebb, meaning that their routine killing of tumor cells in the body had been greatly weakened. The authors emphasized that the degree of immune problems they observed would likely lead to chronic and recurrent infection with herpes viruses.

Even though Klimas and her colleagues singled out the potential of immune dysfunction to lead to the reactivation of herpes viruses in people with CFS, there was by this time little interest in pursuing this link. Early research on EBV and HHV-6 that focused on antibody levels to the viruses had not been persuasive, partly because of the lack of standards in testing.

Thanks to Cheney, interest shot up again in the possibility that a retrovirus was involved in CFS. By then HTLV-1 had gained some notoriety as a possible cause of some rare neuromuscular disorders. One of Cheney's patients had come down with signs of muscular atrophy in his calf. The man had previously developed a variety of symptoms but had tested negative twice for antibodies to HIV. But when Cheney tested him, the test came back positive and was confirmed by a second test. Several repeats of the test, however, came back negative. What on earth was going on? Cheney speculated that the man might have an HTLV-1 infection, possibly its link to muscle problems, accounting for the atrophy in his calf, and the fact that the virus was confounding the HIV antibody test.

This led to more testing at Wistar, and on September 4, 1990, at a medical conference in Kyoto, Japan, DeFreitas presented the results of the study. It showed 82 percent of blood samples from 11 adults with CFS and 74 percent of blood samples from 19 children with CFS had turned up gene segments of a virus similar to both HTLV-1 and HTLV-2, a retrovirus that had been isolated by the Gallo lab from a patient with hairy cell leukemia, a rare form of the disease. None of the 20 controls showed any signs of such viruses in their blood. In none of the experimental subjects or controls were there any signs of HIV.

DeFreitas was very cautious in presenting the results, emphasizing that the data pointed to a strong association between the retroviral segments and CFS. By no means were the researchers claiming to have found the cause of the condition. Much more research was deemed necessary.

Given the complexity of research politics, however, the scientists, including DeFreitas and Cheney, did not refrain from boiling the pot a little. They also indicated that the same viral fragments were found in people in close, non-sexual contact with the experi-

mental subjects. Suggesting the viral agent had been casually transmitted certainly made the news everywhere. But a week later at a
press conference in San Francisco, DeFreitas and Cheney downplayed this aspect of the research, saying the study had not been
designed to explore viral transmission. They had included the result in their report because they were surprised by it. Upon questioning by reporters, they also admitted to being aware of the
powerful public health implications.

Two weeks after the presentation in Japan, Cheney and his
associates began to take a lot of flak from scientists who continued to hold to the theory that CFS resulted from mental anguish.
Strauss, for example, essentially suggested to an audience of scientists in Toronto that the Wistar findings were a crock. "The techniques used to identify the suspect virus are fraught with potential
complications."

Sharp criticism came even from those who believed CFS was
a biological disease. Among them, Scottish researcher John Gow
suggested that the retroviral fragments captured at Wistar were
likely to be genetic sequences issued from human cells. In other
words, Gow was interpreting signs of a retrovirus in CFS much as
the Perth Group scientists interpreted HIV in AIDS.

Still, Cheney was hopeful that he and DeFreitas were on the
right track. They had used three different technologies to reach
their conclusions, and they had tested and retested over more than
two years. They had been careful. Work was ongoing to see if they
could extract the virus, and this could take time. Nonetheless,
Cheney was willing to admit that their suspect virus could turn out
to be unrelated to CFS. The virus might be a marker that becomes
activated due to damaged immunity but does not cause CFS. Some
other, as yet unidentified, virus which destabilizes the immune system could be uncovered.

Cheney would be disappointed. Attempts by others, including
the CDC, to replicate the retroviral research failed, suddenly leaving CFS without any viral explanation. There was, however, another way of looking at CFS that was building in the wings. A far
more controversial, yet innovative way.

*   *   *

Though mild-tempered and thoughtful, soft-spoken John Martin suffers few fools and can appear cranky. When the lanky Australian-born physician became more interested in CFS in the late 1980s, he had access to a large patient population. He then headed the pathology department at the University of Southern California and directed the pathology laboratories at Los Angeles County Hospital, the largest medical teaching institution in the nation.

Rather than an immune dysfunction, CFS looked to him more like an infectious brain disease that could range from extreme to mild. It also struck him that patients diagnosed with CFS had a wide range of neurological symptoms that defied easy cataloging.

His mission, as he saw it, was to uncover the infectious processes that gave rise to this panoply of symptoms. From the start he was aware that any foray into the dynamics of CFS could turn out to be a thankless task. Medicine was far too narrow in its approach to infectious disease; it typically assumed that there was always one viral monster for any particular disease. This was not likely, given that diseases themselves are complex processes in the body and not static slabs of activity that can be margined off from one another. Life was far too sophisticated to support such a simplistic notion of disease.

Martin was well equipped with the latest in lab technology to launch his adventure into CFS and beyond. He also had well-trained, reliable staff at the university and the county hospital. There was no reason why he couldn't take the lead in this matter.

He first wanted a close look at the new herpes virus, HHV-6, that early on had been suggested as a cause of the CFS outbreak at Lake Tahoe. Using PCR to detect and amplify viruses, a technology that he had helped to refine, he at first didn't find any sign of HHV-6 in the blood samples taken by a physician friend from patients with a CFS diagnosis. When he reconfigured the PCR test materials to be less specific for the genetic structure of HHV-6, though, he discovered some readings that indicated something similar to the virus.

Martin then set up the PCR test to amplify all reactions from any of the herpes viruses, including HHV-6. In other words, he was casting the net wider as he fished for signals similar to those sent by the known herpes viruses. Low-level signals were rife when he examined the blood of some of the patients. The immediate implication was that he had tapped into a viral process involved in CFS that had not been previously identified. Maybe even a whole new set of viruses.

He went searching for these atypical virus signals in the cerebrospinal fluid and blood tissue of numerous patients with severe CFS symptoms, notably those with neurological problems, such as memory loss and confusion. As he expected, the signals turned up again and again. What surprised him, however, was the lack of any sign of inflammation in the cerebrospinal fluid biopsies. If there indeed was viral infection, he should also detect signs of an inflammatory process, the sure-proof indication that the patient's immune system had responded to the threat of a virus. Did this mean that he was finding atypical viruses which had somehow changed themselves and were eluding the body's immune system? Stealth viruses? Very likely.

Then came another surprise. By conducting more elaborative tests of CFS-related blood, he detected signals from what appeared to be a virus with genetic ties to both herpes viruses and a retrovirus. Looking at his catch in an electron microscope, he observed that it caused cells to turn foamy-like upon infection. Retroviruses of the spuma family, also known as foamy viruses, could cause such changes to cells. Was this "stealth virus" primarily a spuma? The electron microscope photographs revealing some of its structure suggested it might well be.

With the support of Paul Cheney, to whom he reported his findings, Martin received funding to continue this spuma-related research from a large CFS patient organization (known as the CFIDS—Chronic Fatigue and Immune Dysfunction Syndrome—Association). Before long, he had some evidence of spuma-like viral infection in about half of the 300 CFS patients he had tested. Though the CFS community was excited about his discoveries, mainstream science was not. Martin received publication rejection slips from three major journals: *The Lancet, Journal of the American Medical Association,* and *Annals of Internal Medicine.* In a word, his work was far too preliminary. No, he would not even be allowed to write a letter to the editor. About this time, his troubles really began.

As in any scientific domain, there are well-wishers and there are snipers. Martin began attracting snipers. Some scientists felt he was unwilling to provide immediate answers to questions about the details of his work. This was resented by other CFS researchers who, after all, had the responsibility of keeping CFS science as free from controversy as possible. Even in the best of times, theirs was a major uphill battle. And Martin was becoming more controversial. At a CFIDS-sponsored meeting, one CFS researcher even denounced Martin publicly for being so tight-lipped about his research protocols. The CFIDS Association took careful note. The only way for Martin's work to be seen as credible was if other scientists replicated it. So far no one had done so, partly because they didn't have the exact procedures to follow.

They had reason for concern. Previously, no one had ever cultured viruses from CFS patients. Why was Martin successful? Was the virus really a spuma? And if so, did it really have anything to do with CFS? It could be a dormant virus. Or had he merely produced a laboratory contaminant?

Martin was soon asked to participate in a study that would require him to use his laboratory techniques to differentiate between blood samples from 10 CFS patients and 10 healthy controls. Martin bombed and it didn't play well at CFIDS. In his own defense, he argued that he had used a simpler technique to test the patient samples than he ordinarily used in his lab experiments. Furthermore, Martin believed that because CFS was not a precisely defined disorder with a specific marker, it was wrongheaded to assume that his type of test, which was broadly oriented, would routinely pick up what other people were narrowly defining as CFS. He would later feel foolish that he had allowed himself to be pushed into such a demeaning situation.

Meanwhile, CFIDS lost patience with Martin. There would be no more research money.

Did that fall from grace stop John Martin? Absolutely not. In Washington, D.C., on November 6, 1995, Martin made a gallant effort to convince a federal government science panel to consider his growing public health concerns seriously. He had new viral research to present to the Institute of Medicine that had emerged from his studies of CFS. The data suggested a new and dangerous epidemic was underway that affected many Americans in both subtle and extreme ways. He had already tried repeatedly to get the Centers for Disease Control in Atlanta and the Food and Drug Administration in Bethesda to investigate, but to no avail.

The first slide Martin showed the science panel depicted the crude attempt by a 39-year-old schoolteacher from Palm Springs to draw a clock and a house. This had occurred a year after she noticed she was unable to spell certain words. Her doctor attributed it to stress. A year later, after she found it more difficult to speak and identify things, an MRI scan revealed brain lesions. The next slide showed the results of a brain biopsy; there was no sign of inflammation in the woman's brain tissue. Yet electron microscope studies of her tissue, as seen on the next slide Martin showed, revealed evidence of "atypical structures consistent with herpes viruses."

Slides documenting a second patient's more severe brain problems were similar. She too was a CFS-type patient who had been initially diagnosed as suffering from stress.

So what was this virus? Ongoing research at his two labs had led to a dramatic revelation. The virus was not exactly what he had supposed all along. Unmasking some of the genetic code of the virus had shown it to be very similar to a CMV monkey virus. The final match showed that the CMV core of this stealth virus could only have originated in an African green monkey.

Martin concluded his remarks to the panel this way: "The African green monkey is a major concern with regards to polio vaccines. Therefore, requests have gone repeatedly to CDC, FDA, to begin to look at the issue of live polio vaccines as a potential source of the inadvertent introduction of monkey cytomegalovirus stealth-adapted viruses to the human population."

That ought to get their attention, Martin believed.

What he did not know yet was that monkeys weren't the only animals that might be involved in CFS. An animal much less exotic—in fact, a common household pet—would provide the next clues in the virus hunt.

CAT MYSTERY

Janet of Tulsa, Oklahoma, was 40 years old when she was diagnosed with chronic fatigue syndrome. She was exhausted much of the time, suffered from headaches and a sore throat, and often could barely function. Soon after Janet became ill, she noticed that her cat was lethargic and developing a variety of symptoms, such as urinary tract infections, digestive problems and diarrhea. She also found it very peculiar that her cat could no longer walk normally. Janet began worrying that her cat had also developed a CFS-like illness.

Janet's doctor was Tom Glass, a pathologist and dental surgeon at the University of Oklahoma Health Sciences Center. He had also served as chief dental expert to the medical examiner of the state of Oklahoma. Among his other scientific interests was the transmission of disease, which included novel research on how bacterial, fungal, and viral diseases could be transported by the common toothbrush. Because he enjoyed medical mysteries, he had also become preoccupied with CFS.

Glass had heard other stories like Janet's. Anecdotal accounts were being noted in the CFS literature, and they were the subject of conversation at CFS conferences. If the stories were true, Glass reasoned, they would indeed rank as a significant development in the annals of medicine. With the exception of rabies, there was no evidence of any viral infection transmitted between typical domestic animals and humans.

Glass was curious enough about these stories to develop a questionnaire. Asking a small survey of CFS patients, he wanted to know how many had pets, how they interacted with them, and whether the animals had developed CFS-like symptoms. He ended up with a total of 114 female and 13 male respondents with the condition. The patients came from the community and CFIDS support groups throughout the country. Their average age was 42.

The results of the survey were eye-catching. The vast majority of the patients reported that they had pets (mostly cats and dogs) and interacted with them extensively. Many slept with their animals and often kissed them. They had been bitten or scratched by them. Most of the patients also believed that their pets had developed symptoms that mimicked CFS.

Glass then conducted a second survey which focused on the types of symptoms pets of CFS patients developed. He learned, for example, that they were often lethargic, had urinary tract infections, diarrhea, seizures, tremors, palsies, tail twitching, hind leg dragging, skin rashes, hair loss, inflamed gums, and abdominal distention. Overall, the predominant symptoms appeared to be neurological, much as CFS patients suffered.

Glass knew that he had not conducted a well-controlled study and that he had given the CFS patients a lot of rope to voice opinions about the symptoms of their pets; a portion of these responses were no doubt subjective. On the other hand, he was struck by many of the neurological symptoms that they had listed and felt that he had at least been given valuable food for thought; it certainly seemed possible an infectious agent was being transmitted between CFS patients and their pets. And if there was a link, this would obviously raise serious questions about the closeness that people have with their pets. Some people even allow their pets to lick their dinner forks and spoons and then continue to eat with those utensils. Others allow their pets to lick them on the lips. It troubled Glass that his scientific interests might be intruding on common habits that bind people to their animals.

While he was collecting his data, some CFS patients, including Janet, mentioned to Glass that he could use their very ill pets for study when they died. The idea appealed to him. Perhaps he would find buried in their tissues some sign of infection. In the fall of 1991, he developed a procedure for the autopsies that would be required and received clearance from the university's ethics review board.

Glass conducted his first autopsy on a cat who had died after suffering a variety of neurological symptoms, including recurrent seizures. Drawing blood samples, Glass was sure to take specimens from every part of the cat's body. He processed and preserved tissue and made slides so that he could view them under both light and electron microscopes. Within days he was ready to begin his analysis.

After he placed the first slide of brain tissue in the microscope stage and looked through several lenses, he was surprised. He had expected to find some signs of tissue changes, such as alteration, destruction, inflammation, or scarring. But there was nothing unusual. Nothing. The brain looked normal.

He popped in another slide. Normal. This continued until he viewed the eleventh slide, that of the trigeminal ganglion, a knot of nerve cells on the base of the skull. These cells appeared to be swollen or balloon-like, and had a foamy appearance. There were also groups of lesions within the cells. More brain tissue slides revealed similar patterns. The only time Glass had ever seen something like this before was in immune-deficient children whose bodies had been overwhelmed by herpes virus infections.

Then Glass saw an anomaly in the cells. There was no inflammation—thus no reaction from the immune system. If a virus had caused the changes in the cells, it somehow must have eluded the body's key defenses. This was very peculiar.

He returned to the first few slides from the brain and, keeping the trigeminal ganglion in mind, saw similar changes in other regions such as the hypothalamus, cerebrum, and cerebellum. But again none of the cells were inflamed. The body had not reacted in typical fashion against whatever had attacked these cells.

Glass then turned to a slide of gum tissue. Normally gums are infected with bacteria but not this cat's; the infection appeared to be more viral-like.

Next, Glass began to examine endocrine glands—the adrenals (involved in steroid, sex, and stress hormone control), the pancreas islets (involved in sugar control), the thyroid (involved in metabolism control), and the pituitary (which controls the endocrine system). He found that they all seemed to have an excess of hormonal secretion but also an excess of cells to produce these hormones. Did this mean that the glands were producing sufficient hormone but not releasing it, thus forcing the body to stimulate the production of extra hormone-producing cells? Glass concluded that this was likely the case and that he was observing hormone-producing cells that had been disabled.

This led him to wonder if CFS patients became mentally confused at times and suffered muscle weakness because changes in brain cells resulted in a loss of their full function. As he continued to examine slides of other regions of the body, such as the lymphoid tissue, salivary glands, the respiratory and digestive tracts, the liver, kidney, and blood vessels, he became more convinced that the cat had been attacked by a virus that altered cell function enough to cause a wide range of symptoms.

But Glass knew much more work needed to be done. As exciting as his findings were, the next step was to determine whether there really was some infectious process related to CFS. The next set of experiments would be crucial.

Glass took a blood sample he had drawn from the autopsied sick cat and injected it into a healthy cat. After 48 hours the healthy cat became ill. Its pupils dilated, there was a bloody discharge from the eyes, the lymph nodes got big, and the cat had seizures. A highly detailed autopsy revealed similar findings to the first one. And so did autopsies of other cats injected with what appeared to be infectious blood.

Glass thought he might be sitting on a powder keg. He believed that his research might provide a biological explanation for CFS:

widespread dysfunction in the body triggered by a virus. But he also knew that it would take more than several autopsied cats to convince the scientific world that CFS could be transmitted from humans to animals, never mind vice versa. It was too much of a leap to make without broad research in this direction.

By chance, Glass happened to meet John Martin for the first time at the CFIDS Association meeting. They exchanged stories about life in the CFS trenches, and when Martin learned about the cats, he offered to collaborate with Glass on further research. Martin then sent Glass cells infected with one of his stealth viruses retrieved from a CFS patient so he could inject them into healthy cats.

The five experimental cats developed pretty much the same acute symptoms after 48 hours as the ones that Glass had previously studied. The autopsy results were also remarkably similar. But this time Martin found more information about a possible infectious agent. Studies of brain tissue with the electron microscope revealed the presence of herpes-like viral particles and other bits of what might be virus. And the cats used as controls in the experiment did not get sick, except for very mild symptoms.

Once the initial excitement wore off, reality set in again, even though Glass and Martin had published their results in summer of 1995. The research could only be considered preliminary and would require replication from other research groups before any conclusions could be reached.

John Martin traveled to the East Coast for another chance at convincing the scientific elite that his stealth virus theory should be taken seriously. This time the meeting was sponsored by the National Institute of Allergy and Infectious Diseases, the government's main funding body for research on microbes. It was billed as a "consultation" on the detection of monkey CMV in humans.

This was a critical day for Martin because the NIAID appeared to be his last hope of stirring government interest in his work. The Centers for Disease Control had sat on his funding request for five months before informing him that the genetic decoding of stealth viruses was not a project that met the agency's "needs at this time." The Food and Drug Administration had kept him on hold for seven months before finally advising him that he might try the National Institutes of Health.

Martin knew that he had an uphill battle. It seemed that no one in the scientific establishment wanted to mess with vaccines. Open up this Pandora's box and watch your career go down the chute.

Martin was not one to slam his fist and wave his arms about, but his presentation this day had more of an edge than usual, and his facts were more pointed than those he had aimed at the vaccine panel. First he cited examples chronologically, beginning back in 1940 and running to the present, of how polio vaccines might have become contaminated. There was little new in this review of how the processing of the vaccines appeared to have been corrupted. When Martin completed his vaccine summary, he explained, in heavily technical language, his method of detecting stealth viruses. Then he reviewed in some detail the cat experiment he had conducted with Tom Glass. He was gradually opening up the big picture.

His stealth virus research, he told the NIAID audience, was revealing a broad spectrum of undiagnosed brain diseases that were disabling Americans. Both severe and subtle, psychiatric-like and rheumatic illnesses were at the heart of an epidemic that medicine could not easily detect. The trouble was that medical practice assumed there were clear demarcations of disease rather than overlapping and changing symptoms. Complicating matters further was the need of both doctors and their patients (not to mention government reimbursement agencies) to give names to diseases. Martin argued that this type of diagnostic system had failed miserably to account for debilitating complex processes in the body, and particularly those triggered by a virus that didn't kill cells but appeared to disable them to produce dysfunction. His research showed that stealth viruses could do just that in humans and animals.

Over the years he had detected stealth viruses in patients who were primarily experiencing neurological problems: young children with autism, attention deficit, aggressive behavioral disorders; young adults with schizophrenia, manic depression; adults with impairment of sensory and motor functions; and the elderly diagnosed with Alzheimer's disease.

The brain, he said, was very localized in its functions. A stealth virus could strike anywhere in the brain to cause specific disease.

That was it. The NIAID would either buy it or not. They didn't.

The CDC, which had been monitoring Martin's remarks, felt it necessary to issue a public statement. It concluded this way: "There is no evidence that polio vaccine, or any other vaccine, has been contaminated with a 'stealth' virus. To our knowledge, existence of this virus as suggested by one researcher has not been confirmed by other investigators."

In the body of the brief release, the CDC also made note that there was no confirmation by an independent laboratory that a partial genetic sequence of the "stealth" virus was similar to monkey CMV.

Martin's losses were mounting and his opportunities rapidly dwindling to make a mark with his theory. Another jolt was the ban imposed by the University of Southern California on his lab to test for stealth viruses. This highly political intervention had occurred soon after he had returned to Los Angeles from his presentation in Washington to the Institute of Medicine. Instead he quickly set up shop in a lab he rented in an old hospital. He called his new venture the Center for Complex Infectious Diseases, and vowed to make it into the nation's principal institution for stealth virus research and treatment.

NEW LEASE ON LIFE

Donald Carrigan and Konnie Knox, veterans of coffee-shop science, had been kicking around the idea of starting their own private laboratory for months. Knox had become disenchanted with her job at the hospital. She had found the work environment unfriendly and a staff member not at all shy about claiming credit for ideas developed by others. But then, she wasn't exactly the compliant type in the face of adversity. She had not avoided having some terse interactions with this shameless individual.

Carrigan had left Medical College several months before. Though worried about being out of a job in a university setting, he believed that he and Knox could actually pull off owning their own research lab. They would have to hustle to get contracts, particularly to get the funds to conduct HHV-6 research, but they could initially set some modest goals. And when they got started, they could each draw some income for at least six months. He would be entitled to some unemployment insurance and Knox would keep her job, albeit grudgingly, until perhaps the end of March.

One good omen was a call out of the blue they had received from a philanthropist in Oklahoma who had heard about their work on HHV-6. The man's wife had been diagnosed with chronic fatigue syndrome, and he wanted to help the right sort of projects get started. He wondered whether they might be willing to write up a grant proposal for a CFS study.

Knox considered this invitation another example of how their research path seemed to be one of destiny. They had planned to follow through on their MS work, which had been left languishing, and now they could perhaps look forward to CFS, another neurologically based illness, one badly in need of some solid research. Of course, they had also examined the brain in AIDS and marrow-transplant patients. It all seemed to fit together.

The new laboratory was set up in a converted two-level home across from an apple orchard in a quiet residential neighborhood. Other tenants included an architectural firm and accountants. The lab was actually in a small space that had once been used as a laundry room tucked away by itself steps down from the second-floor hallway. It had a sink and a 220 V outlet. It was just big enough to store a microscope and to set up equipment to perform cell cultures.

In a tiny adjoining room that once had served as an area to fold the laundry was enough room for a desk and some office equipment. The monthly rent for the former laundry suite was two hundred and seventy-five dollars.

Knox had been willing to spend more money, about seventeen thousand per year for a five-year lease when she saw a real laboratory space she loved on sight. Carrigan had stared at her in disbelief, thinking perhaps for the first time that she really was nuts. How could they possibly afford a space like that?

While Knox soldiered on at St. Luke's, Carrigan furnished the laundry suite with used furniture. Filing cabinets and tables cost fifty dollars. An old beast of a microscope with wonderful lenses for seven hundred dollars. A new computer, printer, and fax machine. The cheapest lab supplies he could unearth. And they were ready to do business—at their institute.

"We knew we were taking a huge chance even to set up in this small space," Carrigan remembered. "It was a commitment to get our research going again rather than to look for a job at some company or academic institution. I had never done anything like this before in my life. It was scary."

They signed their first research contract in November with Glaxo. It paid them three thousand dollars to test how the antiviral drug Acyclovir reacted to HHV-6. "It wasn't much, but it was a promising start," Knox said. "So there was good reason to cheer, but I'm a more optimistic individual than Don is."

Hanging over their heads was the terribly slow response by *The Lancet* to accept or reject their manuscript on how lymph nodes in AIDS patients were infested with active HHV-6. They had been waiting for four months; they both felt that this paper was critical to understanding how the immune system in people with AIDS was being destroyed.

On the other hand, Carrigan and Knox knew that there was great hope brewing about new drugs called protease inhibitors. In July, at the Eleventh International AIDS Conference in Vancouver, David Ho had even predicted that the widespread use of these drugs could potentially bring the epidemic to an end. These types of drugs, he said, could eliminate HIV from the body, perhaps in some cases in even one year.

Even to some mainstream HIV researchers, Ho's assessment seemed like a cruel hoax. In their view, he was taking advantage of a population that had been looking for miracles. But most HIV researchers simply bowed to Ho, whose status had shot up rapidly ever since *Time Magazine* in December 1995 had anointed him "Man of the Year." When Ho said strike early and strike hard with combinations of AIDS drugs, referred to as "cocktails," then that's what most doctors began to do.

To Carrigan and Knox, this latest chapter in HIV science didn't make much sense. They vowed to return to their work on AIDS as soon as time, money, and space allowed.

AN ALARMING
OUTBREAK

Donovan Anderson, a large man who speaks softly, is not the type to complain openly about his fate. When pressed, he would concede that he had mixed feelings about the location of his medical practice. He liked running his own medical center on the outskirts of Needles, California. It was rewarding to serve the small community on the Colorado River, where he was known to almost everyone. Yet he often felt stranded in the middle of the wilderness. Fourteen years of doctoring in the desert was more than enough repayment to the Public Health Service for helping him financially through medical school. He hadn't planned on staying for so long, but his risky purchase of the Willow Valley Center had pinned him down. Nor were there any suitors in sight to take it off his hands.

Since February, however, Anderson had been feeling more isolated than usual. The Mohave Valley region had been stricken with an outbreak of mysterious illnesses. Over a period of several months, about two hundred people had shown up at the Willow Valley Medical Center with gastrointestinal upsets, including nausea, vomiting, and diarrhea. He would have dismissed this as a flu-like illness going around, except that fifty of the patients had also developed a range of neurological symptoms, particularly acute episodes of muscular problems, such as right arm or right-side facial weakness. Others suffered sudden bouts of memory loss and sleep disturbance. A few patients found that, upon standing, one of their feet would suddenly lose strength. Typically, the gastrointestinal problems were resolved after two weeks, but many of the patients continued to have what appeared to be chronic residual neurological symptoms.

Anderson noted that the illness spread among live-in family members, relatives, and friends and perhaps even to some family pets, which also suddenly exhibited signs of neurological illness. How so many people in the Mohave Valley region had developed the flu-like symptoms, followed by neurological disorders, was anybody's guess. On the basis of conversations he had with other doctors, including hospital doctors who manned the emergency service in Needles, Anderson estimated that hundreds of additional patients had become ill over the spring and summer. For the most part, the shorthanded medical system in the valley had responded routinely to the outbreak. This response to such a rare outbreak reminded Anderson that the desert was hardly the place for the sophisticated unraveling of a medical mystery. He decided he'd have to try to solve it himself.

The neurological symptoms of his patients bore a striking resemblance to those suffered by people with chronic fatigue syndrome. Prior to the outbreak, he had occasionally seen CFS patients at his medical center. He had not been interested until one day he learned of three patients diagnosed with the condition who had attempted to commit suicide and ended up in the hospital in Needles. They had described their condition as a "living hell" and wanted to exit such a world. Anderson linked up to several CFS chat groups to familiarize himself in greater detail about the range of symptoms of the illness and how doctors addressed them and how patients tried to cope. By the time the outbreak occurred, he had also become acutely aware of the controversies surrounding "yuppie flu." He knew that it would take a lot of convincing to get state health authorities interested in the neurological dysfunction he was seeing in his patients. As expected, after one Arizona epidemiologist returned from his visit to the Mohave Valley, he deemed the neurological symptoms as either nonexistent or likely the signs of peripheral nerve disorders common to diabetes. The matter was therefore officially closed. Maybe for the state of Arizona, but not for Anderson. He would soon team up with an infectious disease specialist aggressively on the lookout for strange medical cases and outbreaks.

John Martin was very pleased. It was a good way to begin a new year. Science conferences were proving to be important avenues to make contact. First Tom Glass from Oklahoma and more recently, last October at the CFS conference in San Francisco, Donovan Anderson from the Mohave Valley, practically in his own backyard. Martin had thought the outbreak was a great opportunity to test for stealth viruses. The symptoms that Anderson had described as CFS-related were, of course, to Martin an oversimplification. He no longer could look at disease in such a narrow fashion. In his view, an infection hitting the brain could cause a wide range of overlapping symptoms depending on where it localized and then spread. Giving the process a name would only obscure its complex and unpredictable nature. His mission was to expose the underlying infectious agents that caused such a broad array of illness. Now, thanks to Anderson's diligent tracking of this outbreak, another milestone in his research had been reached.

Laboratory culture tests that Martin had performed on forty samples of blood he had received from Anderson all showed strong signs of a viral infection having some of the general characteristics of his previously identified stealth virus. The infection caused changes in the microscopic appearance of cells in a culture it grew in, but yet failed to trigger an inflammatory response. In the Mohave samples, however, the cellular changes occurred more quickly than in previous samples. Also, human cells were more strongly affected than the monkey cells he had used before. All the results, including those additionally gleaned from brain-tissue samples from three other patients and a blood sample from a sick dog belonging to a culture-positive couple, were consistent. In other words, there was something that set this stealth virus apart from the other type he had previously cultured, which he believed had originated from African green monkey cytomegalovirus and polio vaccines. The origin of this new virus, the "Mohave stealth virus," would have to be determined through appropriate genetic studies.

Even though these findings could only be considered preliminary, Martin believed, largely on the basis of his lab tests, particularly his studies with the electron microscope showing consistent changes in infected cells, and the sudden eruption of flu-like and neurological symptoms in the Mohave Valley, that a transmissible illness had occurred in that community. Some of the symptoms were similar to those found in CFS patients and in veterans described as having Gulf War Syndrome (GWS).

But equally striking to Martin was that the patients whose blood tested positive for stealth virus infection did not all have similar patterns of disease. Symptoms ranged from mild degrees of neurological disorder of the type often linked with CFS and GWS to more severe illness, including the case of Tina's young son Len, who appeared to be one of the casualties of the outbreak. Martin had tracked the boy's history of deterioration in school and, on the basis of his lab test, believed that Len's body was likely being destroyed by a stealth infection. He regarded the case as further suggestive evidence for his theory that these so-called syndromes were merely part of a continuum of brain diseases ignited by stealth viruses.

Now if only Martin could get the required funding to do the

kind of detailed laboratory follow-up work in the Mohave Valley that might finally arouse the interest of his scientific peers. Population studies would also be important in nailing down the extent of the outbreak. He was even hopeful that a major research assault on stealth viruses might lead to a drug that could inhibit the viral effect. In some of the cell cultures he ran in the lab, he noticed that inhibition of the virus had occurred, possibly through some unidentified factor that had been created in the chemical soup. But without money to conduct further research, he might never be able to extract this inhibitor and prepare it for potential use as a stealth virus drug. The irony here was that Martin understood very well that his best chance of making his case for the existence of stealth viruses was to come up with a cure for stealth viruses.

If Konnie Knox and Donald Carrigan, with their meticulous and well-published research, were having a difficult time of capturing the attention of mainstream scientists, John Martin's hopes were based on what was comparatively incomplete and unverified research. Still, science is unpredictable in its patterns. There is an ongoing dynamic process whereby once seemingly unrelated ideas can eventually link up and prepare the groundwork for new theory and research. Now it was time for Carrigan and Knox to enter the fray again.

BREAKTHROUGH FOR A START-UP LAB?

Seven months had passed since Carrigan and Knox established their laboratory in the laundry room. The cramped quarters where Carrigan had mainly conducted tests showing how a well-known herpes drug could interfere with HHV-6 in the test tube was now merely a satellite for the real laboratory they had set up several miles away.

It was mainly Knox's push that caused the expansion move in February. "Had the decision been left to Don, we might still be banging into one another in the laundry room," Knox explained. Carrigan had gone on unemployment. Feeling vulnerable, he was in no mood to throw money around.

The new acquisition had actually happened by chance. They had been interested in farming out some lab work to a colleague who rented space in a building at a research park, not far from Medical College. When they arrived during a snowstorm in mid-January, they learned that some space was available for an office and lab. Knox immediately began to investigate. Carrigan knew that she had gotten the idea into her head and wasn't about to budge; she loved the facilities. Yet he also understood that if they were ever going to succeed as an independent research team, they wouldn't be able to pull it off in the laundry room. That space had to be viewed as an interim shelter from the storm. So he had agreed to take on the extra cost.

In order to move quickly to acquire the new lab space and avoid tedious paperwork, their friend offered to rent the office and lab spaces and then sublet it to them. Two weeks later, they were in, amazed by their boldness.

They even decided to maintain the laundry room as an office. Knox could use it as a quiet retreat to attend to their business requirements and strategies—more specifically to find ways to pay the bills. For starters, their basic rent was more than $1,500 per month. Then they had to rent freezer space from their friend for their blood and tissue samples. So throw in another couple of hundred. And they had lab and office furniture to buy, a task for the budget-minded Carrigan. Plus the fluorescent microscope they would need, costing $3,000. And so on. They agreed that they would pay most of their bills with credit cards, a decision that struck the worried Carrigan as insane but obviously necessary under the circumstances. Knox took it all more philosophically. After all, flying by the seat of their pants was the only choice they had.

Because scientific enterprise, like most business ventures, requires a chain of command, they gave themselves titles. Knox became Director of Research. Carrigan opted for Director of the Clinical Laboratory. The two directors agreed that their first task was to refine a culture test they had developed at Medical College that could rapidly assess whether HHV-6 was actively infecting human blood and tissue. They hoped this test would catch on and be used widely in patient care and become the cash cow that could finance further HHV-6 studies.

"We both knew there was danger in what we were doing," Carrigan recalled. "It was possible that we could get so caught up in finding ways to fund the lab that our work on HHV-6 would never again get off the ground." They had already lost almost two years of valuable time. Just when their research on bone marrow–transplant patients, people with AIDS, and people with MS had begun to converge and point the way to an understanding of how HHV-6 could ravage the body, they had been forced to put this rapidly developing critical mass of scientific work on hold. Their lab work on the virus had come to almost a complete halt. In his lame-duck year at Medical College, Carrigan, with help from a lab technologist, had managed to complete some preliminary work on detecting active HHV-6 infection in MS brain tissue and to conduct several other small experiments. Yet this was a drop in the bucket compared to the highly productive years he and Knox had put in at Medical College.

In the meantime, they learned that the scientific paper they had written on detecting active HHV-6 in the lymph nodes of people with AIDS would not be published by *The Lancet*. Since they believed that the research represented the smoking gun that HHV-6—and not HIV—was what destroyed lymphoid tissue in AIDS, the rejection by the journal was a blow. The sudden ascendancy of David Ho's HIV theory might have played a role. Ho had portrayed HIV as the destroyer of the immune system's T-4 lymphocytes. It was a theory without actual evidence of cells being destroyed by HIV, but plenty of snowballing agreement that the virus did the job. In these circumstances, AIDS scientists were not about to embrace another virus as a potential co-factor in the process of immune destruction, and certainly not the potential of a common herpes virus doing the damage on its own.

The blow was aggravated when they learned that their paper had been temporarily lost when a key senior reviewer scheduled to read it had taken another job and packed his bags without taking the paper with him. The paper was finally recovered several months later. Such sloppy handling would probably have never happened if Carrigan and Knox had been prominent members of the AIDS establishment. Rather than immediately re-submit their work to another journal, they reasoned that they might be better off to temporarily put this project on the back burner, until such time that it appeared that AIDS research was more open to alternative ideas about how AIDS develops. They would have to be careful now about how they managed their time, money, reputations, and expectations.

Also unsettling to Carrigan and Knox was the fact that other labs were pursuing the HHV-6 link to multiple sclerosis at a time when they themselves could least afford the time and money. For example, a team from Seattle had been first to publish preliminary evidence that HHV-6 was actively involved in brain cells of MS patients where there were signs of destruction. The researchers had concluded that the virus appeared to be associated with the cause or development of the disease, albeit cautioning that any new virus linked to MS had to be viewed with great suspicion, given the long and failed history of scientific attempts to show a viral cause. The paper that Carrigan and Knox had finally published months later on the 27-year-old woman with MS who had served as a control in their AIDS brain research had more or less reached a similar conclusion, only they had used a more detailed test method to identify active HHV-6 infection. Further research during Carrigan's last days at Medical College had been confirming their initial findings.

Their business plan, besides building up their laboratory to serve as a commercial diagnostics lab for HHV-6, was to approach pharmaceutical companies for money to conduct more tests on how drugs could interfere with HHV-6, and also try to convince some funding agencies to give them money for more imaginative research, including work on MS. This was an ambitious plan for two scientists without an important institutional base. "We were probably crazy, but yet determined to carry on," Carrigan remembered.

What didn't help was Carrigan's highly selective social personality. He showed few skills in negotiating for funds, and Knox was becoming worried about his presentations with pharmaceutical companies. He would either become a difficult sour puss or talk on and on about their projects. Worse still, he would tell them what they wanted to know without their having to pay at all. Finally Carrigan and Knox agreed that he would not attend any further sessions. Carrigan, not one bit pleased at this arrangement, sulked at the slightest mention of any social disabilities Knox believed he had. This was not a pleasant time at the new lab. Knox, however, was forever resilient, and believed that if she handled the personal end of the business, there would soon be money in the bank. In only a few short months, she would prove to be right. Thanks to a doctor in Kansas City, she and Carrigan would turn an important corner—in the field of MS.

A patient in that Midwestern city, Diane didn't expect her MS symptoms to go away forever. She was realistic and savvy enough to understand that she was in a battle with this dread disease for life. Still, the early signs were good that she might stave off the worst cycles of the progressive disorder that would rob her of her ability to be active and fully enjoy her life with her husband and their children.

In her thirties, Diane had begun to sense that something wrong was happening to her body. It began with double vision. She began to feel confused at times. She couldn't concentrate. She would lose her balance.

She soon became frightened enough to make a hospital appointment, thinking that perhaps she had a tumor. She didn't. She was diagnosed with MS, a condition she had never even considered and didn't even know much about, except that people often ended up in wheelchairs. She was horrified and felt her life had become hopeless.

The doctor at the hospital told her that her symptoms would subside in time and then it was mostly a matter of waiting to see what would happen next. They would proceed one step at a time. MS was a highly variable disease. Not enough was known about it to determine how an individual would progress.

Diane's second attack, more than a month later, differed from the first. This time she felt tingling and numbness in her hands and feet. She also had the sensation that there was a band or girdle wrapped around her stomach, and she suffered inflammation of her optic nerve. Other nerve-related attacks began to occur every two or three months, each lasting about four to six weeks.

During the first few months of Diane's ordeal, her husband had thoroughly reviewed the types of treatments available to MS patients. He became disheartened when it became apparent to him that there was nothing even approaching a cure. In fact, many of the drugs had highly toxic side effects. But the relapses were com-

ing regularly, and in early September 1997 Diane reluctantly
turned to prednisone, a steroid, for relief. That was shortly before
Dr. Joseph Brewer would meet Konnie Knox at a neurology conference in Toronto. Diane's life would change for the better.

On September 30, at the Thirty-seventh Interscience Conference on Antimicrobial Agents and Chemotherapy, being held in
Toronto, Konnie Knox was presiding over a poster display de-
scribing the preliminary research that she and Carrigan had completed on MS. Poster sessions allow works-in-progress to be
displayed at scientific gatherings, and the participants hope to attract the attention of their scientific peers who stroll down the
aisles inspecting the offerings. To the optimist, some of the posters
might tip the scientific world to what possibly could become the
next bright theory or dramatically effective treatment; to the pes-
simist, posters often represent the bottom of the barrel of what science has to offer, namely redundancy, lack of imagination, and
sham. Knox knew a poster presentation was not the promised
land, since the real action was at the oral presentations where at
least status was usually on display, if not always substance. But she
was happy simply to be in Toronto with wares to show. It was a
miracle that she and Carrigan had made it this far.

The institute was still fighting for its life, but some money had
finally started coming in. They'd gotten a grant from the CFIDS
Association for $80,000 to conduct research on chronic fatigue
syndrome. The National MS Society supplied $25,000 to con-
tinue their work on MS. A $10,000 contract had come from a drug
manufacturer to test a herpes treatment on HHV-6. This was
nowhere near enough to keep above water for very long, but at
least they had a chance of making things work out.

The MS research which the poster unveiled had started back in
Medical College, had then been dropped when Knox was forced to
leave for St. Luke's Medical Center, was periodically revived by occasional bursts of work Carrigan did mainly on his own in his final days at Medical College, was sustained in fits and starts in the
laundry room, and finally, after several months at the research
park, was again revived when the MS money came in. Despite all

the interruptions, Knox believed the final result was a riveting challenge to conventional thinking in the MS field. She was now confident that HHV-6 played a role in the disease.

Posters are not usually formatted with the craven hyperbole of advertisements. Rather, they are highly compressed statements of research results; some of the compressions are simply too daunting to unravel, even for the scientific sophisticate. The Knox-Carrigan poster, however, was simple and to the point, thanks to the clarity of the Knox touch, which had prevailed over the Carrigan touch, which was often much more comprehensive, if not overly dense. Knox had long realized that Carrigan had a need to detail all; a poster would not likely be his main weapon of educating the scientific masses. Her view had won out.

Joe Brewer was walking up and down the poster aisles when he spotted the Knox-Carrigan exhibit. Having a professional interest in viruses, he was immediately curious about HHV-6 and introduced himself to Knox, who was only too happy to provide an overview of the research.

She and Carrigan had tested a total of 24 blocks of central nervous system tissue from seven patients with MS who had died. They detected cells actively infected with HHV-6 in the tissues of three of the seven. In some cases, infected tissue revealed the destruction of myelin, the protective sheath surrounding nerve fibers of the central nervous system. This is the hallmark of MS. Tissues free of demyelination were mostly free of cells infected with HHV-6. As in their other research with AIDS patients and bone marrow–transplant patients, the highlight here again was that destruction of tissue was accompanied by active HHV-6 infection. No destruction, no HHV-6 infection. Knox also explained to Brewer that the seven normal brains they had used as controls showed no signs of cells infected with HHV-6. The same held for tissue from patients who had non-MS types of myelin-destroying disease.

In doing some short-term collaborative work with Steve Jacobson of the National Institutes of Health, Knox and Carrigan had detected a low-level active infection in the lymph nodes of three of four patients with MS. This suggested that an HHV-6 infection could be body-wide, and not only present in the central nervous system of MS patients. Therefore, MS patients could possibly have their peripheral tissues (including blood) tested for active HHV-6 infections. In this way, antiviral drugs could be used in those fighting off an active infection. Knox and Carrigan were indeed in the process of refining their rapid culture blood test that could fill that bill.

Brewer immediately understood what their results might mean for MS patients infected with the virus: the test could be a monitoring tool for assessing the effectiveness of a particular therapy. He was impressed. The science behind this latest round of work appeared solid. Knox and Carrigan seemed to be on to something important. As an infectious disease specialist, he had not treated MS patients; this was a territory largely reserved for neurologists. But maybe that was about to change.

Brewer began thinking of Diane, who had been searching for an effective way to fight her newly diagnosed MS. Maybe she would be interested in taking the blood test to see if she had an HHV-6 infection.

Knox likes the term "serendipity." She believes she and Carrigan are fated to unmask HHV-6 as a major force in disease. The chance meeting with Brewer was another example of the Great Unfolding.

On October 28, Joe Brewer drew a blood sample from Diane, who at the time was still fighting an attack of MS, and sent it to Milwaukee. An eager Knox and Carrigan put it to the test and discovered that Diane was strongly positive for active HHV-6 infection. In fact, there was a massive amount of active virus in her blood.

On November 11, when Diane's symptoms had disappeared, more blood was drawn. This time she turned up negative for HHV-6. On January 23, while Diane was experiencing some sensory loss in her arms and legs, blood tests were again positive for active virus. To Knox and Carrigan, Diane's tests suggested that MS symptoms arose when HHV-6 was reactivated. When the virus returned to dormancy or continued to infect at a very low level, the symptoms would largely resolve. By no means was this proof of anything, but it was certainly an indication of where their research had to focus.

Joe Brewer had the idea that he could begin monitoring patients like Diane on antiviral drugs that were known to interfere with herpes viruses. He was thinking primarily of gancyclovir, which, according to several studies, seemed most likely the best bet to fight HHV-6, at least for the present, until better drugs and drug regimens could be developed.

Brewer, like his newfound colleagues in Milwaukee, knew full well that meddling in the territory of neurologists would not win him many friends in the MS scientific fraternity. He, Knox, and Carrigan would have to do extensive work even to attract attention. On the other hand, should they build up enough of a patient base that responded to therapy directed by their viral monitoring system, this could convince the MS Society and drug companies to help fund clinical trials. Knox and Carrigan were right to believe that HHV-6 would likely get the respect it deserved only when therapies targeting patients with active viral infection showed promise.

BACK TO SQUARE ONE?

While Carrigan and Knox had been gradually extending the evidence of HHV-6's ability to destroy cells, former Man of the Year David Ho's "viral dynamics" had been under heavy review—not only from HIV dissidents but from members of the HIV mainstream itself. As the new year began, more scientific papers were being published that raised serious questions about Ho's theories of eradicating HIV from the body.

Concerns had also been steadily rising about the side effects and overall value of the drug combinations known as "cocktails," doses of AZT combined with so-called protease inhibitors that were said to shut down production of infectious virus. This was not a good time for an HIV establishment that had gone on record as predicting either a possible cure for AIDS within a few years or, at the very least, a powerful therapeutic result, for hundreds of thousands of Americans and millions of people worldwide.

There was also a strong sense of déjà vu in this latest attack on HIV. Early on, one major reason why it was assumed that HIV was a mass killer of T-4 cells had to do with its ability to infect this cell in the laboratory dish. In humans, T-4 cell decline was evident in AIDS, and because of this, the virus was fingered as the culprit.

Even by the late 1980s, though, scientists, then spurred on by Peter Duesberg, had begun to acknowledge that the heavy loss of T-4 lymphocytes that characterized AIDS probably could not be blamed on HIV infecting and then directly wiping out those cells. There didn't seem to be enough of the virus present to attack such an abundance of T-4 cells.

Here were all these HIV proponents trying to tame a virus that showed up very little in the body, presumably late in the disease (being referred to as "latent") and didn't even have the good sense to reveal itself as the destroyer of tissue it was said to infect. What had happened to the fundamentals in science?

Then along came Ho in 1995, revitalizing mainstream AIDS science. According to him, there was so much of HIV swimming around in the blood, as revealed by a laboratory method that "marked" pieces of the virus, that this "viral load" had to be attacked hard and early by combinations of powerful drugs. Ho and his associates reasoned that if HIV replication was stopped, the T-4 cells that were in decline would be capable of bouncing back to normal levels. The HIV-free immune system could reconstitute itself. Hence probably no more AIDS.

Of course, Ho's hope was only theory, and he did caution that his team at the Diamond AIDS Center did not have all the answers. The virus could be lurking in other parts of the body and might therefore be more difficult to destroy. But these caveats were swept aside in the media explosion. Disheartened AIDS patients everywhere were filled with hope. Also swept aside were the flaws in the theory that were immediately exposed by dissidents and members of the HIV fraternity alike. For example, the dissidents pointed out, where was the data that revealed HIV could kill in one manner or another? Was the virus anywhere to be found near destroyed tissue, say, in the lymph nodes? They also criticized the method of establishing viral load, that the amplification technique (known as PCR) supposed to show so much virus in the blood led to an illusion. What was being amplified was not HIV, but bits and pieces of what was only presumed to mark the existence of the virus.

Some members of the AIDS establishment had deep concerns

about the drug cocktails. An example was Jay Levy, a microbiologist at the University of California School of Medicine in San Francisco who has been credited as one of the early HIV pioneers, alongside Montagnier and Gallo. He was worried that Ho had ignored the likelihood that HIV was not primarily in the blood but in tissue "reservoirs" throughout the body. To Levy, these reservoirs served as HIV manufacturing plants. Focusing too much attention on the amount of virus that seeps out of these reservoirs into the blood, as Ho had been doing, was missing the point. The drug treatments were not targeted at the reservoirs but rather the virus in the blood. Ho's approach was therefore overly optimistic.

Levy was particularly concerned about Ho's premise that it was best to give drugs early to even those people infected with the virus but who had no AIDS symptoms. Striking early, as Levy saw it, would only give the virus in those reservoirs a greater opportunity to develop resistance to the drug cocktails. Levy believed that drugs should be given only to those who had AIDS. Plus, these drugs were proving to be highly toxic. Ho had hoped that the drugs would be taken for only a short period of time, but Levy was convinced that once patients got on these drugs, they would probably have to keep taking them for a prolonged period. Levy was convinced that Ho's theory would inevitably be proven wrong. By the time this happened, however, there would be thousands of people taking toxic drugs who didn't yet need to do so.

To dissidents such as Duesberg, Levy had as little evidence for his position as Ho. It was all sheer speculation, based on a host of vague markers that added up to nothing. These premier scientists of the HIV movement, according to Duesberg, were continuing to oversimplify the nature of AIDS. They had no real scientific evidence of HIV causing AIDS.

The new research appeared to cast more doubt on the Ho vision of AIDS. Using new techniques to measure immune cells, scientists came up with disturbing results. Until this time early HIV infection had been associated with a decline in so-called naive T-4 cells (those which had not become mature enough to go into action to fight off invaders). Yet the new tests showed a decline also for naive T-8 cells, other fighters of the immune system. The same decline was noted for mature T-4s and T-8s in later stages of disease. Now, this was odd—indeed a red flag—because HIV was not known to infect T-8s. So why were the T-8s diminishing in detectable numbers as well as the T-4s, which were supposedly being knocked off by HIV? Was this a sign that HIV was not really destroying the T-4s, but that something else was going on in the immune system that led to the decline of both T-4s and T-8s?

One emerging theory proposed that HIV had a profound effect on the entire immune system, blocking production of new immune fighters such as the T-4s and T-8s.

This shift in theory naturally begged the question of why people taking drug cocktails suddenly had more T-4s (and T-8s, as it turned out). One view gave HIV credit for somehow creating the conditions that trapped the immune cells in various tissues such as the lymph nodes and spleen. The drugs were said to ignite a process that began to free up the trapped cells and spit them into the bloodstream where they tallied up as signs of a regenerated immune system.

The bad news here, according to the evolving HIV theory, was that this sudden resurgence of immune cells in the first few weeks of therapy was therefore not evidence of an immune system that was in the throes of restoration. The cells were simply being redistributed as a by-product of drug treatment from one part of the body to another. The troubling implication was that new therapies would have to be designed to shore up the immune system by helping it to reconstitute itself. Attacking HIV was hardly enough to do the job. Unfortunately, AIDS science had put all of its eggs in one basket: the focus had almost entirely been on fighting HIV.

By no means did this sea change in theory affect the strong advocacy for the drug cocktails. To those who had sided with Ho's vision of HIV, the rethinking merely meant that ways would have to be found to boost immunity while the drugs did their job to control the virus as much as possible. The restoration of the immune system would still occur, only now it might take perhaps ten years or even longer.

Meanwhile, reports on the use of the drug cocktails were not very encouraging. Though anecdotes abounded about people rising up like Lazarus from their deathbeds, scientific evidence was still lacking that these drugs could extend patients' lives. The AIDS establishment had come to accept the markers such as "viral load" as a substitute for science that was carefully tracking whether the new drug cocktails actually worked over the longer term. They also accepted the test for viral load as an indication of how someone should be medicated for AIDS, assuming that viral load was an appropriate marker for disease progression. Yet there was no direct evidence to uphold that assumption.

While some reports linked a drop in AIDS deaths to these new drugs, the statistical correlations that drove this data hardly made a strong case. No randomized clinical trials had been conducted, comparing those on the drugs to those who were not. AIDS deaths could be on the decline because of major changes in overall AIDS treatment and reduction of certain behaviors, such as unsafe sex leading to a variety of infections and widespread street drug use that could damage the body. Until the appropriate studies were done, the exact causes could not be tracked.

Furthermore, the therapeutic benefits attributed to these new drug cocktails might not have anything to do with HIV. These types of drugs have antimicrobial properties that could, to varying degrees, target other infections that are common to AIDS. At least some of the improvements seen in patients may be due to this antimicrobial action. But are these benefits enough to outweigh the side effects these drug cocktails have caused?

These side effects began to concern AIDS leaders such as Anthony Fauci, head of the National Institute of Allergy and Infectious Diseases. The numbers of people on the drugs were growing, to date perhaps more than fifty percent of those diagnosed. Patients were watching their bodies change before their very eyes. Faces and limbs began to look wasted, pads of fat were accumulating at the back of the neck, and plasma often looked like cream. Abnormally high counts of blood fats called triglycerides were putting patients at high risk for heart disease. In other cases, patients found the drugs to be too toxic to their blood. Others couldn't afford the fifteen thousand dollars per year required to maintain drug cocktail regimens, or found the complex and highly detailed regimens of 30 pills or more that had to be followed much too daunting.

Carrigan and Knox, while focused on their own continuing HHV-6 research, were not oblivious to the new stirrings in the world of HIV. They began thinking that they should revive their scientific paper on HHV-6's ability to destroy lymph nodes in AIDS patients, the paper that they had sent to *The Lancet* back in the summer of 1996, only a week before Ho presented a case for his HIV theory. Maybe in the new spirit abroad, the paper would get accepted this time around.

Against them stood more than two decades of preoccupation with HIV, almost to the exclusion of other research paths. This was not about to give way in the foreseeable future to alternative explanations of how the immune system could collapse, leaving the body open to an onslaught of infections. Despite its failures, HIV science was proving to be remarkably resilient to a careful re-thinking of its basic premises about the virus and it was equally re-sistant to exploring new avenues of research, including the HHV-6 path being blazed by Knox and Carrigan.

In this context, the lack of effort to try to replicate and advance their work wasn't surprising, even though that neglect of their work could mean that lives were being needlessly lost. It was disturbing that the breadth of their research enterprise, which gave more credibility to their work on AIDS, had not attracted more attention. If more data accumulates showing that HHV-6 was involved, then many years have been wasted in finding appropriate treatments to neutralize it.

BRAIN STATIC

Institute for Viral Pathogenesis, Milwaukee
November 1998

Winter was coming, and just thinking about it made Donald Carrigan uncomfortable. He had never been a snow enthusiast. But these days it didn't take much to make him cranky. He and Knox had to get their feet on the ground financially so that they could get on with their pursuit of science rather than putting so much effort into chasing research grants and doing drone-like lab chores. Carrigan had even been working on weekends to perform lab procedures that any technologist could have easily managed. But there was no extra money for more lab help. "There was just less and less time for us to focus on those endless attempts to get funding for our projects," he lamented. "We wondered how we were going to survive."

Carrigan was also feeling uneasy about his recent encounter with the National Multiple Sclerosis Society. "Don had not been too receptive to the society's concerns that we may have prematurely gone to the press to talk about our MS research," Knox explained, smiling. Both ABC News and *The Boston Globe* had reported on an October 20 poster display on their work in Montreal at the 123rd annual American Neurological Association Meetings. Plus, every now and then Carrigan and Knox would receive an unsolicited request for an interview from newspaper or television reporters, mostly local. One of the senior people at the MS Society suggested to Carrigan that the group, which had given the institute two small pilot research grants, should have been informed well in advance of the Montreal meeting. As a result of those reports, the society had been flooded with calls from patients asking for any information about HHV-6 and potential treatments to combat the virus. Carrigan, while sympathetic to the society's plight, made it clear to the caller that he and Knox had actually sent the society information on their work well in advance. The phone call was only the first round. "There was also a terse exchange of e-mails," Knox added.

At issue was their latest data showing that more than half of a group of 25 MS patients displayed evidence of active HHV-6 infection in their blood. Not one of the 62 healthy people they had studied had been infected. There was also an update on their work with brain tissue. They had already examined samples from 11 patients with MS, and their earlier findings continued to hold: cells actively infected with HHV-6 typically were found in tissue where myelin was being destroyed. An update of their work with lymph node tissue showed that six of nine MS patients were positive for active HHV-6.

Carrigan and Knox had also spoken publicly about clinical work they were beginning with Joe Brewer. Diane had been given gancyclovir and appeared to date to have benefited. Her MS attacks had diminished to the point where she was starting to live a more normal life. They were using their rapid culture blood test to monitor how Diane was responding to treatment. In more than a year of tests, they had learned that when she was on gancyclovir and essentially symptom-free, there was little sign of virus.

Carrigan and Knox were careful to cite this case as merely an example of the type of new research that could be done with MS patients, but the lesson they had learned was that any time a new type of treatment becomes the subject of media attention, there is bound to be a huge response by patients who are desperate for any opportunity to get involved in the experiments. It doesn't matter how much the word *preliminary* is used. The MS Society's position was that everything should be done to prevent such an event from getting out of control, even if it meant holding back on research until such time that it could be presented as verifiable evidence and published in a reputable peer-reviewed journal.

Carrigan did agree somewhat with this point of view. Yet he was annoyed by the thought of any voluntary association such as the National MS Society trying to dictate policy about how research by independent scientists should be made public. He was not about to spend long hours in the lab, only to answer in the end to the concerns of bureaucrats. He had had enough of that kind of meddling at Medical College.

Meanwhile Knox, thinking that any future funding by the MS Society had probably floated down the river, agreed to a breakfast meeting at a posh Milwaukee hotel with an MS representative who happened to be making the rounds of local MS chapters. There she learned the society was actually open to working closely with them in the future. If they truly had found the "trigger" to MS, the society had a list of good researchers that could corroborate the evidence.

This was just the sort of advice that Carrigan didn't want to hear. He had done early work on MS, and he had good contacts in the field. If they needed people to back up their work, he and Knox would make the choices themselves.

As before, it was Knox's mission to carefully steer their research enterprise so that they could both retain their independence and simultaneously reach out to the scientific world for collaboration and funding. Carrigan was certainly not going to assume this role. But this meant less time for her in the lab.

Unlike Donald Carrigan and Konnie Knox, E. Fuller Torrey, a psychiatrist and the executive director of the Stanley Research Foundation, hasn't had to worry about how to pay the monthly rent for his large and well-equipped laboratory. The foundation pays the tab and is wealthy enough to have distributed about 100 grants totaling $20 million for mental health research in 1998.

But like Carrigan and Knox, a fair share of Torrey's own research focuses on brain infection. His studies are aimed at determining whether viruses trigger mental disorders such as schizophrenia, with symptoms such as distortions of reality, language disturbances and fragmentation of thought, and bipolar disorder, characterized by episodes of mania and depression. He is convinced that it is only a matter of time before these illnesses are proven to be mostly virally induced. He believes that herpes viruses, including HHV-6, due to their penchant for nerve tissue, are among the culprits likely involved in the complex process that alters the brain and results in mental illness.

Such an approach has generated controversy in a discipline that for much of this century has been dominated by psychological theory. Even though biological theories have made inroads in the past decade, mainly due to the spectacular rise of brain science, considerable resistance to the notion that viruses can set off mental disturbances still remains. Such breakdowns have traditionally been blamed on bad parenting, early experiences in childhood, genetics, and foul-ups of brain chemicals.

As in AIDS, some of the opposition to viruses inevitably boils down to turf protection. Is it surprising that psychiatrists are not overwhelmed with joy to share their studies of the brain with infectious-disease specialists?

Torrey could care less what the old-timers have to say. He's made a habit of speaking his mind. He began publicly attacking psychiatry back in the mid-1970s for being preoccupied with psychoanalytic views of mental illness and with serving the "worried well" rather than the poor who were ill. Finally, in 1985, after developing a reputation as a maverick, he was demoted from a top-level position at the National Institute of Mental Health. Soon after, he left the government and focused his energies on helping a patient movement to grow into a powerful political force: the National Alliance for the Mentally Ill. Besides becoming a strong voice nationally for appropriate patient care, Torrey also advanced the idea to patients that their mental illness was a brain disease and not some psychological failure.

Based on a variety of suggestive evidence that began building slowly in the 1970s, Torrey came to believe that viruses are at the root of at least some mental illnesses. This was not an entirely new idea. A host of doctors at the turn of the century had hypothesized that infections early in life could play a role in mental development and that schizophrenia might result from chronic infections. Torrey was also intrigued that some people who had come down with the flu during the epidemics of 1918 and 1919 had developed symptoms of schizophrenia and bipolar disorder. Around that time some doctors theorized that schizophrenia was a by-product of brain infection, because some patients recovering from encephalitis exhibited schizophrenic symptoms. With these historical insights in mind, Torrey carefully considered the more modern clues that were surfacing.

He found one clue in the scores of studies that showed that

large numbers of people with either schizophrenia or bipolar disorder were born in the late winter and early spring months. Could viruses, thought to be more active during these months, trigger the illnesses in some manner? What else could account for such a seasonal excess?

Torrey found another clue in the scientific literature published on the variety of immune problems that some schizophrenics develop, including white cell (lymphocyte) abnormalities. In addition, limited test data showed that schizophrenics sometimes had higher than normal levels of antibodies to several viruses, particularly the herpes virus CMV.

Numerous peculiar cases in the literature highlight those individuals who appear to have schizophrenia but end up, after having their cerebrospinal fluid tested for signs of viruses, being diagnosed with a brain infection (encephalitis). Some of these first-glance schizophrenia cases turn out to develop a limp a week after initial symptoms or weakness on the right side of the body. These are conditions known to be caused by herpes viruses.

Even though the overall evidence for a viral process in mental illness was sparse, to say the least, Torrey championed the possibility when writing in psychiatric bulletins about schizophrenia and bipolar disorder. The concept made a lot of sense to him: a virus in brain cells could change the chemistry of the cells. The malfunctioning cells could cause mood changes and distort perception of reality. A chronic infection of brain cells could, for example, stimulate some areas of the brain to cause voices to be heard.

When Torrey accepted an offer in 1990 from the Stanley family from Connecticut to take the helm of a new foundation dedicated to mental illness research, he began thinking of the need to establish a scientific unit that would focus on viruses that might affect the brain. And he felt it was imperative to also develop a brain bank that would collect brains of people with schizophrenia immediately after death. Only then could he study infection by viruses.

There are 44 freezers at the brain bank located on the first floor of a building the research foundation rents from the Uniformed

Services Medical School. The freezers hold whole brains or pieces of brain that will be processed in the laboratory in the form of paper-thin slices for research purposes. About 230 brains have been collected to date and shipped frozen within 48 hours of death to the brain bank by a national network that Torrey established at considerable cost. He pays people large sums to scout for brains of schizophrenics.

Besides sending brain slices (usually without charge) to researchers throughout the world, the brain bank is a steady source of brain tissue for the seven-member research unit Torrey established in the department of pediatrics at Johns Hopkins University School of Medicine in Baltimore. Known as the Stanley Division of Developmental Neurovirology, it is headed by Robert Yolken, a pediatrician and infectious-disease specialist who became inspired by Torrey's belief that viruses play a role in mental illness. Yolken decided that he would shift gears in his own career in pediatric infectious diseases to help determine whether Torrey's views on schizophrenia and bipolar disorder had merit. Both he and Torrey are strongly motivated by the possibility of finding antiviral therapies for people with mental illness.

For Yolken, an unassuming and friendly man, much like Torrey, being on the cutting edge of new thinking in science is very much a roller-coaster ride, but he wouldn't want to be doing anything else. The nature of their research requires probing theoretical ground that remains largely uncharted. And while he easily concedes that strong evidence for the viral theory is still lacking, they nonetheless have experimental results that suggest they are on the right track.

In one major area of research, they have focused their attention on genetic materials in cells and how they might play a role in schizophrenia. In other words, Torrey and Yolken are pursuing the idea that the pieces of DNA that we inherit from our parents, along with the functional genes that carry and encode our life's blueprint, are somehow activated to become viruses (endogenous retroviruses) and produce changes in cells that lead to symptoms of schizophrenia. One trigger to turn on this ancient genetic material is a virus that invades the brain, such as a herpes virus. Another possibility is that the genetic material that awakens to cause damage to brain cells is activated by stress or hormonal factors. Research by Torrey and Yolken has shown that activation of this genetic material, as evidenced by detection of RNA, occurs in about 30 percent of the postmortem brains of schizophrenics. Controls of the same age and gender do not show the activation of this genetic material.

Their research suggests that the exact way that this activated material causes specific disease, say schizophrenia, as opposed to some other brain disease, is highly complex. For example, when the genetic material is activated, it becomes capable of "jumping" to another part of the brain and, acting much like an infection, it reintegrates into a site normally foreign to it. Once again, it waits to be turned on—probably by a virus. When this occurs, the products it releases could alter the cell's function. One scenario that Torrey and Yolken propose is that the particular site in the brain where this occurs dictates the type of disease. They have found, for instance, that in schizophrenics different endogenous retroviruses reintegrate in different areas of the brain from those of individuals with other types of psychiatric problems. A related scenario they propose is that the different endogenous retroviruses that are produced, based upon an individual's genetic inheritance, also affects the type of disease that will be set off and formed in the brain.

What could happen early in life, Torrey and Yolken theorize, is that a virus gets into the brain and eventually establishes a chronic infection that activates endogenous retroviruses, which, in turn, set off illness. They suggest that identical twins who start out with genetically identical brains might differ later on when one, who became infected early in life, develops this chronic brain infection, leading eventually to an illness such as schizophrenia in adolescence. Schizophrenia usually is diagnosed somewhere between the ages of 16 and 30.

Theories aside, Torrey and Yolken are very much encouraged by their pinches of research data. Never mind that their ongoing research thus far represents only a tiny fraction of what needs to be understood about how mental illness develops. To get to the heart of the matter more quickly, perhaps, they figure the parallel route for research will be to test antiviral drugs on people with schizophrenia and other neuropsychiatric illnesses. If this type of medication proves to be effective, it will add considerably to the credibility of their viral pursuits.

Torrey and Yolken's work forms part of a much broader and innovative scientific field that includes questions about how chronic illnesses develop. John Martin is trying to prove the existence of a "stealth virus," the product of combinations of microbes (including a monkey herpes virus contaminating polio vaccines in the 1950s) and genes from human cells. Martin's insistence that brain diseases be viewed as part of a spectrum (triggered by stealth viruses) which sometimes involves some overlapping of symptoms, is much in line with the theoretical model that Torrey and Yolken are pursuing. They have, for example, noted an overlap between schizophrenia and MS. Those with schizophrenia sometimes have immune-system reactions that are common in MS patients, and some with MS have mental disturbances. This relationship goes back to their idea that different brain diseases may have reintegration sites for endogenous retroviruses that have left their original cells and traveled to other parts of the brain. Overlaps might mean that some of the sites are commonly reinfected by the endogenous retroviruses, which are then reactivated and cause mischief in cells. Or some of the same type of endogenous retroviruses that are released from cells are common to both illnesses.

Where does HHV-6 fit into this emerging paradigm? At the very least, the virus may in some instances, such as those already explored by Carrigan and Knox—in bone-marrow transplants, AIDS, and MS—reawaken from dormancy to attack cells it normally preys upon, particularly components of the immune system, thus triggering, or contributing to, disease. Additionally, as Torrey and Yolken suspect, a virus such as HHV-6 may trip the genetic material in cells to set off other harmful processes.

The possibility that a major disease lurks inside the body, waiting to erupt because of the interplay of viruses that live within us, is a frightening proposition.

WONDERS
OF THE BODY

**Calypte Biomedical
Berkeley, California
September 1999**

Howard Urnovitz was on a roll. In just a matter of months he'd had several publications provocative enough to raise him to the level of a biomedical "pacesetter." In a scientific world where more than one deviation from the norm can invite torment, Urnovitz was aware that his latest effort to expound on his views of how chronic disease develops might make his peers uneasy. But that wouldn't stop him. He was confident that he and his colleagues were slowly opening the door to uncharted wonders of the body.

In earlier research he had suggested that multiple vaccines left some Gulf War soldiers with altered immune systems, making them more susceptible to infections dormant in the body waiting to be awakened, including HHV-6. In a recent publication he and his colleagues explored the biological process of how the Gulf War soldiers might have developed symptoms common to chronic fatigue syndrome, such as fatigue, rashes, muscle pain, depression, and respiratory and gastrointestinal problems.

In addition to the vaccines the soldiers were given, Urnovitz considered other kinds of stimuli to which they would likely have been exposed: a variety of chemicals, including pesticides and insect repellents; anti-nerve gas agents; low levels of nuclear and electromagnetic energy; diesel exhaust products; medicines to fight chemical-warfare agents; and toxic smoke fumes from oil-well fires. In the past, whenever such factors had been considered as possible triggers of the syndrome, researchers usually dismissed them as being all over the map; in other words, no one culprit could easily be singled out.

Urnovitz viewed the preoccupation with a single cause as a limited way to understand the dynamics of the body. Chronic diseases were likely to be complex and involve multiple steps: a "trigger" of some sort, such as an environmental toxin or a virus that first causes some physical damage; a "progressor," perhaps a re-activated virus such as HHV-6 (or its related fragments), that further weakens the immune system and causes tissue damage; and "host genes," meaning the body's own genetic material, notably remnants of ancient infections that have become genetically integrated into human cells, that could become activated (as endogenous retroviruses) to contribute to disease.

The tests that he and his colleagues ran on 24 Gulf soldiers suggested that this approach to chronic illness was on the right track. They found that the soldiers had RNA in their serum (the liquid that carries blood cells). RNA, used by DNA to make proteins, is normally not seen outside cells or viruses. The RNA floating in the serum, however, did not come from the basic DNA that everyone inherits from their parents. This RNA originated from new genetic material that had been produced by a reshuffling of genes on the chromosomes when the immune systems of the soldiers came under sustained attack. (One particular chromosome region labeled 22q11.2 was a prime suspect.) In contrast, the fifty controls in the study who had not gone to the Gulf tested negative for RNA in serum. This presence of RNA could therefore be a marker of a breakdown occurring in the normal genetic functioning of the individual. It was the kind of breakdown that could result in chronic illness, including Gulf War syndrome.

Urnovitz believes that the type of chronic illness that eventually emerges is determined by what happens to the new RNA that has been produced by gene reshuffling. If, for example, the RNA makes a protein that the body has never seen before, the immune system could potentially target it as a foreign invader and attack it. This could trigger an autoimmune reaction, a disease process in which the body is essentially attacking its own tissues. Diseases such as multiple sclerosis, lupus, arthritis, and diabetes are among those that are believed to have auto-immune components.

In another publication Urnovitz and Brian Durie, a clinical researcher at Cedars-Sinai Comprehensive Cancer Center in Los Angeles, theorized how a trigger could cause physical damage to cells, which in turn would lead to gene shuffling and to the development of a chronic disease such as cancer. Their focus was on the controversial monkey virus called SV40, which had contaminated polio vaccines given to millions of people from 1955 to 1963 (about 100 million in the U.S. alone). Earlier studies had shown that SV40 could be detected in childhood brain tumors, bone cancers, and mesothelioma, a cancer associated with asbestos exposure. But some researchers involved in these studies recently warned that even though signs of the virus were detected in tumors, there was no definitive proof that SV40 was the cause of these cancers and that more research was necessary.

Urnovitz and Durie reasoned that the role of SV40 in cancer might remain unresolved unless a different approach was taken, one that focused attention on the complex manner in which cells might respond to a viral invader delivered by a vaccine. They theorized that SV40 might trigger gene reshuffling in a fashion similar to the reshuffling triggered by Gulf War vaccines and environmental toxins. SV40 would interact with basic DNA to generate new genes. And if the RNA product of this reshuffling was reinserted back into the original genetic material near so-called cancer genes, the cancer process might become activated. In other words, new, highly concentrated research was necessary in order to determine if SV40 was really a human tumor virus.

Urnovitz then applied the same type of reasoning to AIDS. Here too, an initial series of toxic attacks would damage cells, resulting in a reshuffling of genes. This process in turn could damage immune cells that protect the body from a variety of microbes. Once there was a dip in immunity, a powerful virus like HHV-6 dormant in the body could be reawakened to cause massive destruction.

Could such destruction also work through HHV-6–associated gene reshuffling?

A mysterious case of AIDS suggested that the theory had some merit. Urnovitz-led new research showed that a person could potentially have AIDS without being positive for HIV on the standard antibody tests. The patient was a female farm worker in rural France who was diagnosed with an AIDS-like illness in 1988 and gave birth to a child who died of AIDS-like symptoms. The woman, however, consistently turned up negative for HIV antibodies in her blood. However, what appeared to be an HIV-like virus was identified in the woman several years later.

But when she was given a novel urine test that was able to detect antibodies to certain parts of retroviruses, including retroviral sequences lodged in human cells, she turned up positive. When Urnovitz's team analyzed the segments of what was believed to be part of HIV, they matched them with regions from 14 different chromosomes. In other words, this was preliminary evidence for the reshuffling of genetic material. What is called HIV may be a product of this reshuffling process, which involves genetic material streaming from damaged human cells. It may be only a marker associated with AIDS that indicates cell damage has occurred and that a disease process is likely under way.

Urnovitz was aware of a substantial body of scientific literature, involving hundreds of cases of individuals who had developed an AIDS-like condition, characterized by a variety of infections and low T-cell counts. These numbers now include cases of chronic fatigue syndrome with significant dips in their T-cells. When these non-HIV cases were first reported in 1992, the Centers for Disease Control and Prevention concluded that no new AIDS agent was involved and that these cases did not represent an emerging epidemic. They were more or less written off as unexplained and unimportant and given the name T-Lymphocytopenia, Idiopathic CD4-Positive (ICL for short).

Urnovitz views these so-called ICL cases as highly important and perhaps a key to understanding AIDS. So far he hasn't had much luck encouraging traditional HIV researchers to test out his theory of reshuffling genes. One exchange of e-mail with a prominent HIV researcher recently ended in the charge that Urnovitz and his colleagues probably are producing a laboratory artifact, not a real result, whenever they use the urine test in their research. The writer even suggested to Urnovitz that any further exchange of e-mail would likely be unproductive. Urnovitz responds to this type of dismissiveness of new ideas with a grimace. He believes that he has gathered sufficient preliminary data of the complexity of AIDS to be concerned that the HIV mainstream has made a major error.

Facing up to complexity in any chronic illness might quickly dampen enthusiasm for a cure, especially the likelihood that a magic bullet can be found to stop disease progression in its tracks. What Urnovitz is truly proposing is a way of understanding how intimately our changing inner environment is dynamically linked to the changing outer world we live in. There is no escape from change swirling inside and outside of us. The body will react powerfully—and unpredictably—when there is sustained assault. In the end, there is no such thing as immunity to life itself. There is only a spectrum of health or illness.

Is there a way to reduce the rate at which chronic disease progresses? Urnovitz recommends that a major focus be placed not on the triggers of disease, since they are many and are often difficult to isolate, but rather on the insidious factors that enhance the damage already set in motion. He is referring here to infectious agents, but he has in mind primarily a virus that can pack a powerful punch when it reawakens in the body: HHV-6, or its related gene fragments.

Have scientists stumbled on a new way of thinking about viral infections and chronic diseases? Are those who are tracking HHV-6, particularly Knox and Carrigan, also revealing signs of genetic rearrangement triggered by the virus?

If science hopes to unlock the mystery of how chronic diseases occur, it seems likely that an emphasis will have to be placed on better understanding how viruses might help to orchestrate changes in the body's genetic programs.

THE TANGLED
ROAD AHEAD

Before Konnie Knox walks to the podium to give her invited talk to a group of New York City microbiologists, she must solve the problem of the slide projector. The projectionist hasn't shown up, and there do not appear to be enough parts available to make the machine work. This is not good news because Knox has grown accustomed to explaining the details of her HHV-6 work with Donald Carrigan while pointing to various numbers and graphs on a series of slides. A slide presentation is a common, if not indispensable, feature of scientific meetings.

Several of her friends in the audience try to fiddle with the projector as some members of the academy become restless and begin to glance repeatedly at their watches. Finally, someone opens a small box and finds the missing parts, including the remote control for the speaker. With relief the evening's hostess gives Knox a short, almost perfunctory introduction, and the lights are dimmed.

Knox does not attempt to warm up the 60 people in the audience with the usual tributes and gentle humor. She gets right to the subject. Click, slide one, a sum-up of the key features of HHV-6. By this time few are looking at the petite blond woman at the podium who is speaking in a surprisingly strong voice. Rather, all eyes are following her light pointer on the screen. They will remain glued to the dancing red spot for the duration of the presentation.

She has come a long way from the early, shaky days of her research with Carrigan at Medical College. This is now a confident individual who could easily lead other scientists in a new, bold direction. This is a woman who, with Donald Carrigan, committed herself to a life in scientific research by renting a former laundry suite in order to launch a private laboratory when all else seemed to be failing. She never gave up.

The battle, of course, still must go on. The institute in its present quarters is showing some life, now that a surprise backer, a man whose wife struggles with MS, has stepped in to help out on the financial and legal side of things. But even though there is now money in the bank, more HHV-6 research in the pipeline, and a growing need for extra staff and space, Knox knows full well that she and Carrigan are at a turning point. Either their message about this killer virus continues to get out in a way that will compel the scientific community to pay attention, or they will eventually have to fold their tent due to lack of interest and funding. This is one reason why Knox has been giving a series of talks, often leaving Carrigan in Milwaukee to go about the business of heading the institute's research. "We're at the stage where we now must educate scientists and the public about this virus, or there won't be much hope of finding ways to counter its impact in the population," she says.

Knox has reached the stage in her research with HHV-6 that her face tightens when she is asked about the prospects for the institute and her fight to get more scientists interested in studying the virus. "You can say that things are looking up in some ways because we're still alive and kicking in the lab, but how much longer that will be I really don't know," she says with a hint of defiance.

Even so, Knox gives the impression that she and Carrigan are in it for the long haul, no matter what new obstacles they will have to face. Over dinner with her, I remarked that they eventually might even become so successful that they'll become part of the mainstream and adopt some of the arrogant, know-it-all attitudes.

"I wonder what you and Don will be like when you have three or four floors of lab space."

"Oh, we'll probably be pretty much the same if that should ever happen," she said, her face guarded. That's an underlying feature of her expressions: being guarded against surprise. She lives with the fear that there is much to lose if you don't protect your turf.

"I've seen Bob Gallo recently," I told Knox.

"Oh, yeah, what did he have to say?"

"He said that you and Don have done great work on HHV-6."

"Did he really say that?"

"Yes, he did, and he also said that if he were a young scientist today, he'd spend his time working on HHV-6."

That drew a laugh from Knox. "He abandoned HHV-6, and he says he'd be spending his time on it?"

"He says he had personal reasons for abandoning it."

When asked why he has neglected HHV-6 research after promoting the virus for a couple of years as a likely co-factor in AIDS, Gallo explained that about the time that he felt he was making some inroads in HHV-6, aggressive congressional investigators were looking into reports that he had mismanaged his scientific work on HIV. There simply was not enough time to pursue HHV-6 as much as he would have liked, given his ongoing HIV research.

Gallo spoke very generously about what Knox and Carrigan had accomplished, but he also emphasized that they work in too much obscurity to obtain any funding. "They have clearly shown that HHV-6 is a powerful pathogen," Gallo said. "If they were headliners at a major university, it would make a huge difference."

In other words, if they had the kind of financial backing and prestige he had, there would be a lot of interest in HHV-6. Gallo, having left NCI, is now ensconced in smart new digs in Baltimore at the University of Maryland and continues to focus almost all his attention on HIV, hoping to bring in new treatments and a vaccine.

There is a world of difference between the "institute" in Milwaukee and the "institute" in Baltimore. The facility that Gallo works in so far has more than 8.5 million dollars in funding support for 1999. Its 152-member staff has 31 patent filings to its credit and has published 196 peer-reviewed articles since opening day.

But the virology institute that Gallo directs has only a small unit devoted to HHV-6. The unit has been researching whether the presence of HHV-6 DNA in serum and of HHV-6 antibody levels of a certain type correlate with a worsening of MS symptoms. But even Paola Secchiero, the scientist who heads that research, failed to get government funding recently for an HHV-6 project. (Gallo concedes the proposal was improperly targeted to attract funding even though it is under his watch.) He, however, vows to soon step into the breach and do his part to remedy the rather unfortunate lack of funding for HHV-6 research.

"I wish he would do something like that, if he really could," Knox said, a wicked smile broadening.

"You don't believe him?"

"I'd like to believe him."

She won't divulge her views on AIDS science. For one thing, she and Carrigan do keep an open mind on HIV. But their research on HHV-6 has taught them that this virus often appears to be doing what HIV is supposed to be doing in different parts of the body such as in the lymphoid tissue and brain tissue: it is killing cells. Their research also suggests that HIV may not always be necessary as a companion to HHV-6 when the herpes virus is destroying tissue. But even suggesting this in writing would raise the hackles of HIV researchers. In fact, some AIDS scientists compare any questioning of the HIV hypothesis, as it currently stands, to denial of the Holocaust. With such emotions running strong in AIDS science, why take a chance of boldly presenting alternative hypotheses?

This is one reason why Knox and Carrigan do not wish to be associated with any of the AIDS dissidents, such as Peter Duesberg, who has discovered what it means to try to swim upstream. He is barely surviving at Berkeley primarily because of the kindness of strangers who send in donations. A recent effort on his behalf to bring in money landed a grant of $400,000 from a philanthropist. But this won't be enough to sustain research for very long.

Duesberg continues to criticize the AIDS establishment on HIV, still believing that it should not be characterized as the cause of the epidemic. His alternative explanation, that street drugs and pharmaceuticals are the culprits in AIDS, has not made strong inroads publicly, although in recent publications in non-mainstream journals, Duesberg has offered enough of an argument to be taken seriously by some. But once an individual is marginalized, there is generally little concern or respect shown for his data or theories. Given the establishment's access to media, journals and symposia, it becomes easy for the defenders of the faith to brush off any challenger. It's generally believed that he had his opportunity several years back to beat back the tide of HIV theory, and he failed to do so.

Meanwhile, in Australia there is a steady drumbeat of anti-HIV theory slowly seeping into the world consciousness, largely by way of the Internet. HIV has never been isolated. It's wrong to speak of HIV particles because there is no solid proof that they exist. An HIV test, you say? Really? Which one? Worldwide there are at least ten sets of criteria for defining what is positive on the "Western blot" test, the one that is presumed to be so much better than the "Elisa" test. Being positive in some hospitals or nations is not seen as being antibody positive in others. What is going on here? they ask. Are we headed for a major embarrassment—an unprecedented scandal—once this issue hits the right nerve?

Knox and Carrigan, while aware of the issues, want no active part of this often hostile debate. They can't see that it holds any immediate consequences, one way or the other, for their scientific work on HHV-6. They will continue to document their findings and make an all-out effort to get the data out. Then their scientific peers can judge for themselves. If in the end, they won't make a dent in current HIV theory, then it won't be for lack of solid HHV-6 data. And furthermore, HHV-6 is much more than a virus that appears to play a powerful role in AIDS. They have tracked it step by step through a host of other trouble that it causes in the bone marrow, lungs, and brain tissue of transplant patients. It's active in the blood of up to 70 percent of people with chronic fatigue syndrome that are tested. And Knox and Carrigan also find it active in the blood and brain tissue of people with MS.

In recent months, it has been their MS work that's attracted the most attention. At a workshop on MS in Brighton, England, in late August, a group of scientists interested in MS focused some of their attention on the need to hasten research on HHV-6. Knox had been invited to give a talk on her MS research with Carrigan and infectious disease physician Joe Brewer in Kansas City, Missouri. "It was very heartening to see that there was a consensus that work should go on in this area," Knox said, adding that she expects the same will occur at a meeting scheduled for late October in Venice, Italy. "I get the feeling that maybe something will come of this, and we can move on some of the research we've been hoping to do, especially trials that look at treatments for HHV-6."

As her talk and the clicking of slides before the academy audience continues, Knox lays out the research on HHV-6 and MS in a highly efficient and easy-to-follow manner. Carrigan has contributed to this presentation by creating graphics that are eye-catching and simple in detail. The audience quietly takes it all in.

Knox emphasizes that Joe Brewer's patient, Diane, whom they now have followed for close to two years, has less active HHV-6 infection because of treatment with the antiviral drug gancyclovir. They have also discovered that the drug works best if it is administered intravenously rather than in tablet form. But Diane is far from cured; she shows more signs of MS as time goes on. Knox believes better drug treatment will become crucial for MS patients in order to control HHV-6. "We badly need clinical trials to be funded to understand how we can keep the virus in check," she concludes.

The audience keeps Knox busy with a flurry of technical questions about HHV-6 and about its role in MS for about 20 minutes until the host says it's time to end the proceedings and lock up the academy building for the night.

In the wings sits Howard Urnovitz, who happened to have arrived that same day to give a talk at New York University and had heard from friends about the talk. Knox, who has met him previously, is surprised to see him.

"I came here from California just to hear you," he says, always the comedian.

"Sure, you did," Knox replies.

"I think we can do some work together," Urnovitz probes gently. "I've become more interested in HHV-6 recently because I think it can help explain a lot about how chronic disease develops."

Urnovitz believes that Knox and Carrigan are researching a time bomb. Besides its cell-killing potential, according to Urnovitz, HHV-6 also can lead to a reshuffling of genes that send out their messenger chemicals to other parts of the body where they trigger disease processes. Urnovitz believes that HHV-6 can become highly involved in such a process. He wants to join Knox and Carrigan in experiments that would determine whether this actually occurs.

Knox smiles at the suggestion that they work together, offering no clear commitment. She and Carrigan must manage their time very carefully, even if it means holding back on intriguing ideas that might lead to important payoffs. One never knows where these adventures might lead. She will discuss Urnovitz's enthusiastic offer with Carrigan.

Urnovitz leaves the academy already planning how they might conduct the experiments.

On the way to her hotel, Knox seems a little sad. She says she misses her family and does not particularly like the traveling life. She is not even that keen on going to Venice, which she has never seen. "If this keeps up, I'll be doing less and less science, and I don't want that to happen."

I mention to her that travel goes with the territory, and she nods in agreement. I sense that she realizes that her scientific life—and Carrigan's—is only beginning.

Bibliography

Ablashi, D.V., Ablashi, K.L., Kramarsky, B., and others. Viruses and chronic fatigue syndrome: current status. *Journal of Chronic Fatigue Syndrome* 1(2), 1995, p. 3.

Ablashi, D.V., and others. Human B-lymphotropic virus (human herpesvirus-6). *Journal of Virological Methods* 21, 1988, p. 29.

Ablashi, D.V., Bernbaum, J., DiPaolo, J.A. Human herpesvirus 6 as a potential copathogen. *Trends in Microbiology* 3(8), 1995, p. 324.

Ablashi, D.V., Kreuger, G.R.F., Salahuddin, S.Z., eds. *Human Herpesvirus 6: Epidemiology, Molecular Biology, and Clinical Pathology.* Amsterdam: Elsevier, 1992.

Ablashi, D.V., Salahuddin, S.Z., Joseph, S.F., Imam, F., Lusso, P., and Gallo, R.C. HBLV (or HHV-6) in human cell lines. *Nature* 329, 1987, p. 207.

Adler, S.P., McVoy, M., Chou, S., Hempfling, S., and others. Antibodies induced by a primary cytomegalovirus infection react with human herpesvirus 6 proteins. *Journal of Infectious Diseases* 168(5), 1993, p. 1119.

Agut, H. Puzzles concerning the pathogenicity of human herpesvirus [editorial]. *New England Journal of Medicine* 329(3), 1993, p. 203.

Agut, H., and others. In vitro sensitivity of human herpesvirus 6 to antiviral drugs. *Research in Virology* 140, 1989, p. 219.

Akashi, K., Eizuru, Y., Sumiyoshi, Y., Minematsu, T., and others. Brief report: severe infectious mononucleosis-like syndrome and primary human herpesvirus 6 infection in an adult. *New England Journal of Medicine* 329(3), 1993, p. 168.

Ando, Y., Kakimoto, K., Ekuni, Y., Ichijo, M. HHV-6 infection during pregnancy and spontaneous abortion [letter]. *The Lancet* 340, 1992, p. 1289.

Asano, Y., Nakashima, T., Yoshikawa, T., Suga, S., Yazaki, T. Severity of human herpesvirus-6 viremia and clinical findings in infants with exanthem subitum. *Journal of Pediatrics* 118, 1991, p. 891.

Asano, Y., Yoshikawa, T., Kajita, Y., Ogura, R., and others. Fatal encephalitis/encephalopathy in primary human herpesvirus-6 infection. *Archives of Disease in Childhood* 67, 1992, p. 1484.

Asano, Y., Yoshikawa, T., Suga, S., Hata, T., and others. Simultaneous occurrence of human herpesvirus 6 infection and intussusception in three infants. *Pediatric Infectious Disease Journal* 10, 1991, p. 335.

Asano, Y., Yoshikawa, T., Suga, S., Nakashima, T., and others. Reactivation of herpesvirus type 6 in children receiving bone marrow transplants for leukemia [letter]. *New England Journal of Medicine* 28, 1991, p. 324.

Aubin, J.T., Agut, H., Collandre, H., Yamanishi, K., and others. Antigenic and genetic differentiation of the two putative types of human herpes virus 6. *Journal of Virological Methods* 41(2), 1993, p. 223.

Aubin, J.T., Collandre, H., Candotti, D., Ingrand, D., and others. Several groups among human herpesvirus 6 strains can be distinguished by Southern blotting and polymerase chain reaction. *Journal of Clinical Microbiology* 30, 1992, p. 2524.

Balachandra, K., Bowonkiratikachorn, P., Poovijit, B., Thattiyaphong, A., and others. Human herpesvirus 6 (HHV-6) infection and exanthem subitum in Thailand. *Acta Paediatrica Japonica*, 33, 1991, p. 434.

Barnes, D. Mystery disease at Lake Tahoe challenges virologists and clinicians. *Science* 234, 1986, p. 541.

Barre-Sinoussi, F., Chermann, J.C., Rey, F. Isolation of a retrovirus from a patient at risk for Acquired Immune Deficiency Syndrome (AIDS). *Science* 220, 1983, p. 868.

Biberfeld, P., Kramarsky, B., Salahuddin, S.Z., and Gallo, R.C. Ultrastructure characterization of a new B-lymphotropic DNA virus (HBLV) isolated from patients with lymphoproliferative disease. *Journal of the National Cancer Institute* 79, 1987, p. 933.

Biberfeld, P., Petren, A.L., Eklund, A., and others. Human herpesvirus-6 (HHV-6, HBLV) in sarcoidosis and lymphoproliferative disorders. *Journal of Virological Methods* 26, 1988, p. 133.

Bookchin, D., Schumacher, J. The Lonely Crusade of Walter Kyle. *Boston Magazine,* June 1997, p. 58.

Buchwald, D., and others. A chronic illness characterized by fatigue, neurologic and immunologic disorders and active human herpesvirus type 6 infection. *Annals of Internal Medicine* 116(2), 1992, p. 103.

Buchwald, D., and others. A chronic, "postinfectious" fatigue syndrome associated with benign lymphoproliferation, B-cell proliferation, and active replication of human herpesvirus-6. *Journal of Allergy and Clinical Immunology* 10, 1990, p. 335.

Buchwald, D., Cheney, P.R., Peterson, D.L., Henry, B., and others. A chronic illness characterized by fatigue, neurologic and immunologic disorders, and active human herpesvirus type 6 infection. *Annals of Internal Medicine* 116(2), 1992, p. 103.

Buchwald, D., Hooton, T.M., Ashley, R.L. Prevalence of herpesvirus, human T-lymphotropic virus type 1, and treponemal infections in Southeast Asian refugees. *Journal of Medical Virology* 38(3), 1992, p. 195.

Burd, E.M., Carrigan, D.R. Human herpesvirus 6 (HHV-6)-associated dysfunction of blood monocytes. *Virus Research* 29(1), 1993, p. 79.

Burd, E.M., Knox, K.K., Carrigan, D.R. Human herpesvirus-6-associated suppression of growth factor-induced macrophage maturation in human bone marrow cultures. *Blood* 81(6), 1993, p. 1645.

Campadelli-Fiume, G., Guerrini, S., Liu, X., Foa-Tomasi, L. Monoclonal antibodies to glycoprotein B differentiate human herpesvirus 6 into two clusters, variants A and B. *Journal of General Virology* 74 (10), 1993, p. 2257.

Carrigan, D.R. Bone marrow suppression by human herpesvirus-6: comparison of the A and B variants of the virus. *Blood* 86, 1995, p. 835.

Carrigan, D.R. Human herpesvirus-6 and bone marrow transplantation. *Blood* 86, 1995, p. 294.

Carrigan, D.R., Drobyski, W.R., Russler, S.K., Tapper, M.A., and others. Interstitial pneumonitis associated with human herpesvirus-6 infection after marrow transplantation. *The Lancet* 338, 1991, p. 147.

Carrigan, D.R., Harrington, D., Knox, K.K. Subacute leukoencephalitis caused by cns infection with human herpesvirus-6 manifesting as acute multiple sclerosis. *Neurology* 47, 1996, p. 145.

Carrigan, D.R., Knox, K.K. Human herpesvirus 6 (HHV-6) isolation from bone marrow: HHV-6-associated bone marrow suppression in bone marrow transplant patients. *Blood* 84, 1994, p. 3307.

Casserta, M.T., and others. Neuroinvasion and persistence of human herpesvirus 6 in children. *Journal of Infectious Diseases* 170:1586, 1994.

Challoner, P., and others. Plaque-associated expression of human herpesvirus 6 in multiple sclerosis. *Proceedings of the National Academy of Sciences* 92, 1995, p. 7444.

Clerici, M., and others. Immune responses to antigens of human endogenous retroviruses in patients with acute or stable multiple sclerosis. *Journal of Neuroimmunology* 99, 1999, p. 173.

Collandre, H., Aubin, J.T., Agut, H., Bechet, J.M., Montagnier, L. Detection of HHV-6 by the polymerase chain reaction. *Journal of Virological Methods* 31, 1991, p. 171.

Cone, R.W., and others. Human herpesvirus 6 in lung tissue from patients with pneumonitis after bone marrow transplantation. *New England Journal of Medicine* 329:156, July 15, 1993, comment in: *New England Journal of Medicine* 1993 July 15, 329(3):203-4.

Cone, R.W., Hackman, R.C., Huang, M.L., Bowden, R.A., and others. Human herpesvirus 6 in lung tissue from patients with pneumonitis after bone marrow transplantation. *New England Journal of Medicine* 329(3), 1993, p. 156.

Cone, R.W., Huang, M.L., Ashley, R., Corey, L. Human herpesvirus 6 DNA in peripheral blood cells and saliva from immunocompetent individuals. *Journal of Clinical Microbiology* 31(5), 1993, p. 1262.

Cone, R.W., Huang, M.L., Hackman, R.C., Corey, L. Coinfection with human herpesvirus 6 variants A and B in lung tissue. *Journal of Clinical Microbiology* 34, 1996, p. 877.

Corbellino, M., Lusso, P., Gallo, R.C., Parravicini, C., and others. Disseminated human herpesvirus 6 infection in AIDS [letter]. *The Lancet* 342, 1993, p. 1242.

Daibata, M., and others. Inheritance of chromosomally integrated human herpesvirus 6 DNA. *Blood* 94 (5), 1999, p. 1545.

Dalgleish, A.G., and Weiss, R.A., eds. *HIV and the New Viruses*, 2nd ed. San Diego: Academic Press, 1999.

De Vinci, C., Levine, P.H., Pizza, G., Fudenberg, H.H., Orens, P., Pearson, G., Viza, D. Lessons from a pilot study of transfer factor in chronic fatigue syndrome. *Biotherapy* 9(1-3), 1996, p. 87.

Dewhurst, S., McIntyre, K., Schnabel, K., Hall, C.B. Human herpesvirus 6 (HHV-6) variant B accounts for the majority of symptomatic primary HHV-6 infections in a population of U.S. infants. *Journal of Clinical Microbiology* 31(2), 1993, p. 416.

Di Luca, D., Secchiero, P., Bovenzi, P., Rotola, A., and others. Reciprocal in vitro interactions between human herpesvirus-6 and HIV-1 Tat. *AIDS* 5, 1991, p. 1095.

Dolcetti, R., and others. Frequent detection of human herpesvirus 6 DNA in HIV-associated lymphadenopathy. *The Lancet* 344, 1994, p. 543.

Doniger, J., Muralidhar, S., Rosenthal, L.J. Human cytomegalovirus and human herpesvirus 6 genes that transform and transactivate. *Clinical Microbiology Reviews* 12(3), 1999, p. 367.

Downing, R.G., and others. Isolation of human lymphotropic herpesviruses from Uganda. *The Lancet* ii, 1987, p. 390.

Drobyski, W.R., Dunne, W.M., Burd, E.M., Knox, K.K., and others. Human herpesvirus-6 (HHV-6) infection in allogeneic bone marrow transplant recipients: evidence of a marrow-suppressive role for HHV-6 in vivo. *Journal of Infectious Diseases* 167(3), 1993, p. 735.

Drobyski, W.R., Eberle, M., Majewski, D., Baxter-Lowe, L.A. Prevalence of human herpesvirus 6 variant A and B infections in bone marrow transplant recipients as determined by polymerase chain reaction and sequence-specific oligonucleotide probe hybridization. *Journal of Clinical Microbiology* 31(6), 1993, p. 1515.

Drobyski, W.R., Knox, K.K., Majewski, D., Carrigan, D.R. Brief report: Fatal encephalitis due to variant B human herpesvirus-6 infection in a bone marrow-transplant recipient. *New England Journal of Medicine* 330(19), 1994, p. 1356.

Duesberg, P.H. AIDS acquired by drug consumption and other noncontagious risk factors. *Pharmacology and Therapeutics* 55, 1992, p. 201.

Duesberg, P.H. Foreign-protein-mediated immunodeficiency in hemophiliacs with and without HIV infection. *Genetica* 95, 1995, p. 51.

Duesberg, P.H. Human immunodeficiency virus and acquired immunodeficiency syndrome: correlation but not causation. *Proceedings of the National Academy of Sciences* 86, 1989, p. 755.

Duesberg, P.H. *Inventing the AIDS Virus*. Washington: Regnery, 1996.

Duesberg, P.H. Retroviruses as carcinogens and pathogens: expectations and reality. *Current Advances in Cancer Research* 47, 1987, p. 1199.

Duesberg, P., Rasnick, D. The AIDS dilemma: drug diseases blamed on a passenger virus. *Genetica* 98, 1998, p.1.

Durie, B.G.M., Urnovitz, H.B. Cell and molecular biology of simian virus 40: implications for human infections and disease. *Journal of the National Cancer Institute* 91 (13), 1999, p. 1166.

Ensoll, B., Lusso, P., Schlachter, F., and others. Human herpes virus-6 increases HIV-1 expression in co-infected T cells via nuclear factors binding to the HIV enhancer. *EMBO Journal* 8, 1989, p. 3019.

Fairfax, M.R., Schacker, T., Cone, R.W., Collier, A.C., Corey, L. Human herpesvirus 6 DNA in blood cells of human immunodeficiency virus-infected men: correlation of high levels with high CD4 cell counts. *Journal of Infectious Diseases* 169(6), 1994, p. 1342.

Fillet, A.M., Raguin, G., Agut, H., Boisnic, S., and others. Evidence of human herpesvirus 6 in Sjogren syndrome and sarcoidosis [letter]. *European Journal of Clinical Microbiology and Infectious Diseases* 11(6), 1992, p. 564.

Fisher, B.L. Shots in the Dark. *Next City Summer*, 1999, p. 33.

Flamand, L., Gosselin, J., Stefanescu, I., Ablashi, D., Menezes, J. Immunosuppressive effect of human herpesvirus 6 on T-cell functions: suppression of interleukin-2 synthesis and cell proliferation. *Blood* 85, 1995, p. 1263.

Flamand, L., Stefanescu, I., Ablashi, D.V., Menezes, J. Activation of the Epstein-Barr virus replicative cycle by human herpesvirus 6. *Journal of Virology* 67(11), 1993, p. 6768.

Fox, R.I., Luppi, M., Kang, H.I., Ablashi, D., Josephs, S. Detection of high levels of human herpes virus-6 DNA in a lymphoma of a patient with Sjogren's syndrome [letter]. *Journal of Rheumatology* 20(4), 1993, p. 764.

Frenkel, N., and others. Isolation of a new herpesvirus from human CD4-positive T cells. *Proceedings of the National Academy of Sciences* 87, 1990, p. 748.

Fukuda, K., Straus, S.E., Hickie, I., and others. The chronic fatigue syndrome: a comprehensive approach to its definition and study. *Annals of Internal Medicine* 121, 1994, p. 953.

Furukawa, M., Yasukawa, M., Yakushijin, Y., Fujita, S. Distinct effects of human herpesvirus 6 and human herpesvirus 7 on surface molecule expression and function of CD4+ T cells. *Journal of Immunology* 152(12), 1994, p. 5768.

Gallo, R.C. A personal perspective on HIV-AIDS research. *Journal of Human Virology* 2(1) 1999, p. 8.

Gallo, R.C. *Virus Hunting*. New York: Basic Books, 1991.

Gallo, R.C., and others. Frequent detection and isolation of cytopathic retroviruses (HTLV-III) from patients with AIDS and pre-AIDS. *Science* 224, 1984, p. 500.

Gallo, R.C., and others. Isolation of human T-cell leukemia virus in acquired immune deficiency syndrome (AIDS). *Science* 220, 1983, p. 865.

Geng, Y.Q., Chandran, B., Josephs, S.F., Wood, C. Identification and characterization of a human herpesvirus 6 gene segment that transactivates the human immunodeficiency virus type 1 promoter. *Journal of Virology* 66, 1992, p. 1564.

Gobbi, A., and others. Human herpesvirus 6 (HHV-6) causes severe thymocyte depletion in SCID-hu Thy/Liv mice. *Journal of Experimental Medicine* 189(12) 1999, p. 1953.

Gopal, M.R., Thomson, B.J., Fox, J., Tedder, R.S., Honess, R.W. Detection by PCR of HHV-6 and EBV DNA in blood and oropharynx of healthy adults and HIV seropositives. *The Lancet* 335, 1990, p. 1598.

Gompels, U.A., Carrigan, D.R., Carss, A.L., Arno, J. Two groups of human herpesvirus 6 identified by sequence analyses of laboratory strains and variants from Hodgkin's lymphoma and bone marrow transplant patients. *Journal of General Virology* 74(4), 1993, p. 613.

Gompels, U.A., Luxton, J., Knox, K.K., Carrigan, D.R. Chronic bone marrow suppression in immunocompetent adult by human herpesvirus 6 [letter]. *The Lancet* 343, 1994, p. 735.

Gompels, U.A., Nicholas, J., Lawrence, G., et al. The DNA sequence of human herpesvirus-6: structure, coding content, and genome evolution. *Virology* 290, 1995, p. 29.

Gupta, S., Vayuvegula, B. A comprehensive immunological analysis in chronic fatigue syndrome. *Scandinavian Journal of Immunology* 33, 1991, p. 319.

Hagiwara, K., Komura, H., Kishi, F., Kaji, T., Yoshida, T. Isolation of human herpesvirus-6 from an infant with Kawasaki disease [letter]. *European Journal of Pediatrics* 151(11), 1992, p. 867.

Hagiwara, K., Yoshida, T., Komura, H., Kishi, F., Kaji, T. Isolation of human herpesvirus-6 from an infant with Kawasaki disease [letter]. *European Journal of Pediatrics* 152(2), 1993, p. 176.

Hall, C.B., Long, C.E., Schnabel, K.C., Caserta, M.T., and others. Human herpesvirus-6 infection in children. A prospective study of complications and reactivation. *New England Journal of Medicine* 331(7), 1994, p. 432.

Herbert, A.M., Bagg, J., Walker, D.M., Davies, K.J., Westmoreland, D. Seroepidemiology of herpes virus infections among dental personnel. *Journal of Dentistry*, 23(6), 1995, p. 339.

Hill, A.E., Hicks, E.M., Coyle, P.V. Human herpes virus 6 and central nervous system complications [letter]. *Developmental Medicine and Child Neurology* 36(7), 1994, p. 651.

Ho, D.D. Time to hit HIV, early and hard. *New England Journal of Medicine* 333, 1995, p. 450.

Ho, D.D., and others. Rapid turnover of plasma virions and cd4 lymphocytes in HIV-1 infection. *Nature* 373, 1995, p. 123.

Hoffmann, A., Kirn, E., Kuerten, A., Sander, C., and others. Active human herpesvirus-6 (HHV-6) infection associated with Kikuchi-Fujimoto disease and systemic lupus erythematosus (SLE). *In Vivo 5*, 1991, p. 265.

Horvat, R.T., Parmely, M.J., Chandran, B. Human herpesvirus 6 inhibits the proliferative responses of human peripheral blood mononuclear cells. *Journal of Infectious Diseases* 167(6), 1993, p. 1274.

Horvat, R.T., Wood, C., Balachandran, N. Transactivation of human immunodeficiency virus promoter by human herpesvirus 6. *Journal of Virological Methods* 63, 1989, p. 970.

Huang, L.M., and others. Human herpesvirus 6 associated with fatal haemophagocytic syndrome. *The Lancet* 336, 1990, p. 60.

Huang, L.M., Lee, C.Y., Chen, J.Y., Lee, P.I., and others. Roseola infantum caused by human herpesvirus-6: report of 7 cases with emphasis on complications. *Journal of the Formosa Medical Association* 90, 1991, p. 579.

Huang, L.M., Lee, C.Y., Lee, P.I., Chen, J.M., Wang, P.J. Meningitis caused by human herpesvirus-6. *Archives of Disease in Childhood* 66, 1991, p. 1443.

Inoue, N., Dambaugh, T.R., Pellett, P.E. Molecular biology of human herpesviruses 6A and 6B. *Infectious Disease Agents* 2(6), 1993, p. 343.

Johnson, H. *Osler's Web: Inside the Labyrinth of the Chronic Fatigue Syndrome Epidemic.* New York: Crown, 1996.

Jones, C.M., Dunn, H.G., Thomas, E.E., Cone, R.W., Weber, J.M. Acute encephalopathy and status epilepticus associated with human herpes virus 6 infection. *Developmental Medicine and Child Neurology* 36(7), 1994, p. 646.

Josephs, S.F., Ablashi, D.V., Salahuddin, S.Z., Jagodzinski, L.L., and others. Identification of the human herpesvirus 6 glycoprotein H and putative large tegument protein genes. *Journal of Virology* 65, 1991, p. 5597.

Josephs, S.F., and others. Genomic analysis of the human B-lymphotropic virus (HBLV). *Science* 234, 1986, p. 601.

Josephs, S.F., Henry, B., Balachandran, N., Strayer, D., and others. HHV-6 reactivation in chronic fatigue syndrome [letter]. *Archives of Disease in Childhood* 337, 1991, p. 1346.

Kadakia, M.P., and others. Human herpesvirus 6: infection and disease following autologous and allogeneic bone marrow transplantation. *Blood* 87(12), 1996, p. 5341.

Kanegane, H., Ochiai, H., Shiraki, K. Human herpesvirus 6 as a causal agent of the first febrile episode after birth [letter]. *Pediatric Infectious Diseases Journal* 12(2), 1993, p. 171.

Kawaguchi, S., Suga, S., Kozawa, T., Nakashima, T., and others. Primary human herpesvirus-6 infection (exanthem subitum) in the newborn. *Pediatrics* 90(4), 1992, p. 628.

Kion, T.A., and Hoffmann, G.W. Anti-HIV and anti-anti-MHC antibodies in alloimmune and autoimmune mice. *Science* 253, 1991, p. 1138.

Knox, K.K., and others. Fulminant human herpesvirus six encephalitis in a human immunodeficiency virus-infected infant. *Journal of Medical Virology* 45(3), 1995, p. 288.

Knox, K.K., and others. Progressive immunodeficiency and fatal pneumonitis associated with human herpesvirus 6 infection in an infant. *Clinical Infectious Diseases* 20, 1995, p. 406.

Knox, K.K., Carrigan, D.R. Active HHV-6 infection in the lymph nodes of HIV infected patients: in vitro evidence that HHV-6 can break HIV latency. *Journal of AIDS and Human Retroviruses*, 1996.

Knox, K.K., Carrigan, D.R. Active human herpesvirus 6 (HHV-6) infection of the central nervous system in patients with AIDS. *Journal of AIDS and Human Retroviruses* 9, 1995, p. 69.

Knox, K.K., Carrigan, D.R. Disseminated active HHV-6 infections in patients with AIDS. *The Lancet* 343, 1994, p. 577.

Knox, K.K., Carrigan, D.R. HHV-6 and CMV pneumonitis in immunocompromised patients [letter]. *The Lancet* 343, 1994, p. 1647.

Knox, K.K., Carrigan, D.R. In vitro suppression of bone marrow progenitor cell differentiation by human herpesvirus 6 infection. *Journal of Infectious Diseases* 165(5), 1992, p. 925.

Koide, W., Ito, M., Torigoe, S., Ihara, T., Kamiya, H., Sakurai, M. Activation of lymphocytes by HHV-6 antigen in normal children and adults. *Viral Immunology*, 11(1), 1998, p. 19.

Kondo, K., Kondo, T., Okuno, T., Takahashi, M., Yamanishi, K. Latent human herpesvirus 6 infection of human monocytes/macrophages. *Journal of General Virology* 72, 1991, p. 1401.

Kondo, K., Nagafuji, H., Hata, A., Tomomori, C., Yamanishi, K. Association of human herpesvirus 6 infection of the central nervous system with recurrence of febrile convulsions. *Journal of Infectious Diseases* 167(5), 1993, p. 1197.

Krueger, G.R.F., and others. Antibody prevalence to HBLV (human herpesvirus-6) and suggestive pathogenicity in the general population and in patients with immune deficiency syndromes. *Journal of Virological Methods* 21, 1988, p. 125.

Krueger, G.R.F., and others. Clinical correlates of infection with human herpesvirus-6. *In Vivo* 8, 1994, p. 457.

Krueger, G.R.F., and others. Persistent fatigue and depression in patient with antibody to human B-lymphotropic virus. *The Lancet* ii, 1987, p. 36.

Krueger, G.R.F., Sander, C., Hoffmann, A., Barth, A., and others. Isolation of human herpesvirus-6 (HHV-6) from patients with collagen vascular diseases. *In Vivo* 5, 1991, p. 217.

Kusuhara, K., Ueda, K., Okada, K., Miyazaki, C., and others. Do second attacks of exanthem subitum result from human herpesvirus 6 reactivation or reinfection? *Pediatric Infection* 10, 1991, p. 468.

Lau, Y.L., Peiris, M., Chan, G.C., Chan, A.C., Chiu, D., Ha, S.Y. Primary human herpes virus 6 infection transmitted from donor to recipient through bone marrow infusion. *Bone Marrow Transplantation*, 21(10), 1998, p. 1063.

Lawrence, G.L., and others. Human herpesvirus 6 is closely related to human cytomegalovirus. *Journal of Virology* 64 (1), 1990, p. 287.

Levine, P.H., Ablashi, D.V., Saxinger, W.C., Connelly, R.R. Antibodies to human herpes virus-6 in patients with acute lymphocytic leukemia. *Leukemia* 6(11), 1992, p. 1229.

Levine, P.H., Ebbesen, P., Ablashi, D.V., Saxinger, W.C., and others. Antibodies to human herpes virus-6 and clinical course in patients with Hodgkin's disease. *International Journal of Cancer* 51(1), 1992, p. 53.

Levine, P.H., Jahan, N., Murari, P., Manak, M., Jaffe, E.S. Detection of human herpesvirus 6 in tissues involved in sinus histiocytosis with massive lymphadenopathy (Rosai-Dorfman disease). *Journal of Infectious Diseases* 166(2), 1992, p. 291.

Levy, J.A. *HIV and the Pathogenesis of AIDS*, 2nd ed. Washington: American Society for Microbiology, 1998.

Levy, J.A. Surrogate markers in AIDS research. Is there truth in numbers? *Journal of the American Medical Association* 276, 1996, p. 161.

Linnavuori, K., Peltola, H., Hovi, T. Serology versus clinical signs or symptoms and main laboratory findings in the diagnosis of exanthem subitum (roseola infantum). *Pediatrics* 89(1), 1992, p. 103.

Lipkin, W.I., and Hornig, M. Neurovirology: microbes and the brain. *The Lancet* 352 (suppl 4), 1998, p. 21.

Ljungman, P. Herpes virus infections in immunocompromised patients: problems and therapeutic interventions. *Annals of Internal Medicine* 25(4), 1993, p. 329.

Lunel, F., Agut, H., Robert, C., Huraux, J.M., and others. Is human herpes virus 6 (HHV-6) infection associated with posttransfusion hepatitis? [letter]. *Transfusion Science* 31, 1991, p. 872.

Luppi, M., and others. Integration of human herpesvirus 6 genome in human chromosomes. *The Lancet* 352, 1998, p. 1707.

Luppi, M., Barozzi, P., Maiorana, A., and others. Human herpesvirus 6: a survey of presence and distribution of genomic sequences in normal brain and neurological tumors. *Journal of Medical Virology* 47, 1995, p. 105.

Luppi, M., Barozzi, P., Maiorana, A., Marasca, R., Torelli, G. Human herpesvirus 6 infection in normal human brain tissue [letter]. *Journal of Infectious Diseases* 169(4), 1994, p. 943.

Luppi, M., Barozzi, P., Marasca, R., Ceccherini-Nelli, L., Torelli, G. Characterization of human herpesvirus 6 genomes from cases of latent infection in human lymphomas and immune disorders [letter]. *Journal of Infectious Diseases* 168(4), 1993, p. 1074.

Luppi, M., Marasca, R., Barozzi, P., Artusi, T., Torelli, G. Frequent detection of human herpesvirus-6 sequences by polymerase chain reaction in paraffin-embedded lymph nodes from patients with angioimmunoblastic lymphadenopathy and angioimmunoblastic lymphadenopathy-like lymphoma. *Leukemia Research* 17(11), 1993, p. 1003.

Lusso, P., and others. Diverse tropism of human B-lymphotropic virus (human herpesvirus 6). *The Lancet* ii, 1987, p. 743.

Lusso, P., and others. Infection of delta/gamma T lymphocytes by human herpesvirus 6: transcriptional induction of CD4 and susceptibility to HIV infection. *Journal of Experimental Medicine* 181, 1995, p. 1303.

Lusso, P., and others. In vitro cellular tropism of human B-lymphotropic virus (human herpesvirus-6). *Journal of Experimental Medicine* 167, 1988, p. 1659.

Lusso, P., and others. Productive infection of CD4-positive and CD8-positive mature human T cell populations and clones by human herpesvirus 6. *Journal of Immunology* 147, 1991, p. 685.

Lusso, P., Ensoli, B., Markham, P.D., and others. Productive dual infection of human CD4+ T lymphocytes by HIV-1 and HHV-6. *Nature* 337, 1989, p. 370.

Lusso, P., Gallo, R.C. HHV-6 and CMV pneumonitis in immunocompromised patients [letter]. *The Lancet* 343, 1994, p. 1647.

Lusso, P., Gallo, R.C. Human herpesvirus 6 in AIDS. *The Lancet* 343, 1994, p. 555.

Lusso, P., Gallo, R.C. Human herpesvirus 6 in AIDS. *Immunology Today* 16(2), 1995, p. 67.

Lusso, P., Malnati, M., De Maria, A., Balotta, C., and others. Productive infection of CD4+ and CD8+ mature human T cell populations and clones by human herpesvirus 6. Transcriptional down-regulation of CD3. *Journal of Immunology* 147, 1991, p. 685.

Lusso, P., Malnati, M., Garzino-Demo, A., Crowley, R.W., Long, E.O., Gallo, R.C. Infection of natural killer cells by human herpesvirus 6. *Nature* 362, 1993, p. 458.

Lusso, P., Secchiero, P., Crowley, R.W. In vitro susceptibility of Macaca nemestrina to human herpesvirus 6: a potential animal model of coinfection with primate immunodeficiency viruses. *AIDS Research and Human Retroviruses* 10(2), 1994, p. 181.

Marshall, G.S., Gesser, R.M., Yamanishi, K., Starr, S.E. Chronic fatigue in children: clinical features, Epstein-Barr virus and human herpesvirus 6 serology and long term follow-up. *Pediatric Infectious Diseases Journal* 10, 1991, p. 287.

Martin, M.E., Nicholas, J., Thomson, B.J., Newman, C., Honess, R.W. Identification of a transactivating function mapping to the putative immediate-early locus of human herpesvirus 6. *Journal of Virology* 65, 1991, p. 5381.

Martin, W.J. Cellular sequences in stealth viruses, *Pathobiology* 66, 1998, p. 53.

Martin, W.J. Detection of RNA sequences in cultures of a stealth virus isolated from the cerebrospinal fluid of a health care worker with chronic fatigue syndrome. *Pathobiology* 65, 1997, p. 57.

Martin, W.J. Genetic instability and fragmentation of a stealth viral genome. *Pathobiology* 64, 1996, p. 9.

Martin, W.J. Severe stealth virus encephalopathy following chronic-fatigue-syndrome-like illness: clinical and histopathological features. *Pathobiology* 64, 1996, p. 1.

Martin, W.J. Simian cytomegalovirus-related stealth virus isolated from the cerebrospinal fluid of a patient with bipolar psychosis and acute encephalopathy. *Pathobiology* 64, 1996, p. 64.

Martin, W.J. Stealth virus epidemic in the Mohave Valley. *Pathobiology* 65, 1997, p. 51.

Martin, W.J. Stealth virus isolated from an autistic child. *Journal of Autism and Developmental Disorders* 25, 1995, p. 223.

Martin, W.J., and others. African green monkey origin of the atypical cytopathic stealth virus isolated from a patient with chronic fatigue syndrome. *Clinical Diagnostic Virology* 4, 1995, p. 93.

Martin, W.J., Glass, R.T. Acute encephalopathy induced in cats with a stealth virus isolated from a patient with chronic fatigue syndrome. *Pathobiology* 63, 1995, p. 115.

Martin, W.J., Zeng, L.C., Ahmed, K., Roy, M. Cytomegalovirus-related sequences in an atypical cytopathic virus repeatedly isolated from a patient with the chronic fatigue syndrome. *American Journal of Pathology* 145, 1994, p. 440.

Medveczky, P.G., Friedman, H., Bendinelli, M., eds. *Herpesviruses and Immunity*. New York: Plenum Press, 1998.

Merelli, E., Sola, P., Faglioni, P., Poggi, M., and others. Newest human herpesvirus (HHV-6) in the Guillain-Barre syndrome and other neurological diseases. *Acta Neurologica Scandinavia* 85(5), 1992, p. 334.

Merlino, C., Giacchino, F., Segoloni, G.P., Ponzi, A.N. Human herpesvirus-6 infection and renal transplantation [letter]. *Transplantation* 53(6), 1992, p. 1382.

Mookerjee, B.P., Vogelsang, G. Human herpes virus-6 encephalitis after bone marrow transplantation: successful treatment with gancyclovir. *Bone Marrow Transplantation* 20(10), 1997, p. 905.

Moore, P. Herpesvirus 6 might trigger multiple sclerosis. *The Lancet* 350, 1997, p. 1685.

Mullis, K.B. *Dancing Naked in the Mind Field*. New York: Pantheon, 1998.

Newkirk, M.M., Watanabe, Duffy, K.N., Leclerc, J., Lambert, N., Shiroky, J.B. Detection of cytomegalovirus, Epstein-Barr virus and herpes virus-6 in patients with rheumatoid arthritis with or without Sjogren's syndrome. *British Journal of Rheumatology* 33(4), 1994, p. 317.

Okada, K., Ueda, K., Kusuhara, K., Miyazaki, C., and others. Exanthem subitum and human herpesvirus 6 infection: clinical observations in fifty-seven cases. *Pediatric Infectious Disease Journal* 12(3), 1993, p. 204.

Okuno, T., Higashi, K., Shiraki, K., and others. Human herpesvirus 6 infection in renal transplantation. *Transplantation* 49, 1990, p. 519.

Okuno, T., Mukai, T., Baba, K., Ohsumi, Y., and others. Outbreak of exanthem subitum in an orphanage. *Journal of Pediatrics* 119, 1991, p. 759.

Okuno, T., Takahashi, K., Balachandra, K., and others. Seroepidemiology of human herpesvirus 6 infection in normal children and adults. *Journal of Clinical Microbiology* 27, 1989, p. 651.

Oldstone, B.A. *Viruses, Plagues and History*. New York: Oxford University Press, 1998.

Ostrom, N. *America's Biggest Coverup*. New York: TNM, 1993.

Ostrom, N. *What Really Killed Gilda Radner: Frontline Report on the Chronic Fatigue Syndrome Epidemic*. New York: TNM, 1991.

Pantaleo, G. How immune-based interventions can change HIV therapy. *Nature Medicine* 3, 1997, p. 483.

Papadopulos-Eleopulos, E. Reappraisal of AIDS: is the oxidation caused by the risk factors the primary cause? *Medical Hypothesis* 25, 1988, p. 151.

Papadopulos-Eleopulos, E., and others. A critical analysis of the HIV-T4-cell-AIDS hypothesis. *Genetica* 95, 1995, p. 5.

Papadopulos-Eleopulos E., Turner, V.F., Papadimitriou, J.M. Is a positive western blot proof of HIV infection?. *Bio/Technology* 11, 1993, p. 696.

Papadopulos-Eleopulos, E., Turner, V.F., Papadimitriou, J.M., Bialy, H. AIDS in Africa: distinguishing fact and fiction. *World Journal of Microbiology and Biotechnology* 11, 1995, p. 135.

Parker, C.A., Weber, J.M. An enzyme-linked immunosorbent assay for the detection of IgG and IgM antibodies to human herpesvirus type 6. *Journal of Virological Methods* 41(3), 1993, p. 265.

Patnaik, M., Komaroff, A.L., Conley, E., Ojo-Amaize, E.A., Peter, J.B. Prevalence of IgM antibodies to human herpesvirus 6 early antigen (p41/38) in patients with chronic fatigue syndrome. *Journal of Infectious Diseases*, 172, 1995, p. 1364.

Perron, H., Garson, J.A., Bedin, F., and others. Molecular identification of a novel retrovirus repeatedly isolated from patients with multiple sclerosis. *Proceedings of the National Academy of Sciences* 94, 1997, p. 7583.

Pietroboni, G.R., and others. Antibody to human herpesvirus 6 in saliva. *The Lancet* i, 1988, p. 1059.

Pitalia, A.K., Liu-Yin, J.A., Freemont, A.J., Morris, D.J., Fitzmaurice, R.J. Immunohistological detection of human herpes virus 6 in formalin-fixed, paraffin-embedded lung tissues. *Journal of Medical Virology* 41(2), 1993, p. 103.

Popovic, M., and others. Detection, isolation and continuous production of cytopathic retroviruses (HTLV-III) from patients with AIDS and pre-AIDS. *Science* 224, 1984, p. 497.

Portolani, M., and others. Primary infection by HHV-6 variant B with a fatal case of hemophagocytic syndrome. *New Microbiology* 20(1) 1997, p. 7.

Prezioso, P.J., and others. Fatal dissemination infection with human herpesvirus-6. *Journal of Pediatrics* 120 (6), 1992, p. 921.

Qavi, H.B., Green, M.T., Lewis, D.E., Hollinger, F.B., Pearson, G., Ablashi, D.V. HIV-1 and HHV-6 antigens and transcripts in retinas of patients with AIDS in the absence of human cytomegalovirus. *Investigative Ophthalmology and Visual Science* 36, 1995, p. 2040.

Rawlinson, W.D., Hueston, L.C., Irving, W.L., Cunningham, A.L. Cytomegalovirus meningoencephalitis in healthy adults with coincident infection by human herpesvirus type 6. *Australian and New Zealand Journal of Medicine* 22(5), 1992, p. 504.

Razzaque, A., Knox, K.K., Carrigan, D.R., Varricchio, F. Human herpesvirus-6-associated malignant lymphoma in a bone marrow transplant recipient, *Clinical Diagnoses in Virology* 2, 1994, p. 305.

Reeves, W.C., Pellett, P.E., Gary, H., Jr. The chronic fatigue syndrome controversy [letter]. *Annals of Internal Medicine* 117(4), 1992, p. 343.

Reux, I., Fillet, A.M., Agut, H., Katlama, C., and others. In situ detection of human herpesvirus 6 in retinitis associated with acquired immunodeficiency syndrome [letter]. *American Journal of Ophthalmology* 114(3), 1992, p. 375.

Root-Bernstein, R. *Rethinking AIDS:The Tragic Cost of Premature Consensus.* New York: Free Press, 1993.

Rosenfeld, C.S., Rybka, W.B., Weinbaum, D., Carrigan, D.R., and others. Late graft failure due to dual bone marrow infection with variants A and B of human herpesvirus-6. *Experimental Hematology* 23, 1994, p. 626.

Russler, S.K., Tapper, M.A., Knox, K.K., Liepins, A., Carrigan, D.R. Pneumonitis associated with coinfection by human herpesvirus 6 and Legionella in an immunocompetent adult. *American Journal of Pathology* 138, 1991, p. 1405.

Salahuddin, S.Z., and others. Isolation of a new virus, HBLV, in patients with lymphoproliferative disorders. *Science* 234, 1986, p. 596.

Sarngadharan, M.G., and others. Antibodies reactive to human T-lymphotrophic retroviruses (HTLV-III) in the serum of patients with AIDS. *Science* 224, 1984, p. 506.

Schirmer, E.C., Wyatt, L.S., Yamanishi, K., Rodriguez, W.J., Frenkel, N. Differentiation between two distinct classes of viruses now classified as human herpesvirus 6. *Proceedings of the National Academy of Sciences* 88, 1991, p. 5922.

Schonnebeck. M., Krueger, G.R., Braun, M., Fischer, M., and others. Human herpesvirus-6 infection may predispose cells to superinfection by other viruses. *In Vivo* 5, 1991, p. 255.

Schupbach, J., and others. Serological analysis of a subgroup of human T-lymphotrophic retroviruses (HTLV-III) associated with AIDS. *Science* 224, 1984, p. 503.

Secchiero, P., Carrigan, D.R., Asano, Y. and others. Detection of human herpesvirus 6 in plasma of children with primary infection and immuno-suppressed patients by polymerase chain reaction. *Journal of Infectious Diseases* 171, 1995, p. 273.

Shanavas, K.R., Kala, V., Vasudevan, D.M., Vijayakumar, T., Yadav, M. Anti-HHV-6 antibodies in normal population and in cancer patients in India. *Journal of Experimental Pathology* 6(1-2), 1992, p. 95.

Shenton, J. *Positively False: Exposing the Myths Around HIV and AIDS.* London: I.B. Tauris, 1998.

Shiraki, K., Mukai, T., Okuno, T., Yamanishi, K., Takahashi, M. Physico-chemical characterization of human herpesvirus 6 infectivity. *Journal of General Virology* 72, 1991, p. 169.

Singh, N., Carrigan, D.R. Human herpesvirus-6 in transplantation: an emerging pathogen. *Annals of Internal Medicine* 124, 1996, p. 1065.

Singh, N., Carrigan, D.R., and others. Variant B human herpesvirus-6 associated febrile dermatosis with thrombocytopenia and encephalopathy in a liver transplant patient. *Transplantation* 60, 1995, p. 1355.

Singh, N., Carrigan, D.R., Gayowski, T., Marino, I.R. Human herpesvirus-6 infection in liver transplant recipients: documentation of path-ogenicity, *Transplantation* 64, 1997, p. 674.

Sloots, T.P., Mackay, I.M., Carroll, P. Meningoencephalitis in an adult with human herpesvirus-6 infection [letter]. *Medical Journal of Australia* 159(11-12), 1993, p. 838.

Sobue, R., Miyazaki, H., Okamoto, M., Hirano, M., and others. Fulminant hepatitis in primary human herpesvirus-6 infection [letter]. *New England Journal of Medicine* 324, 1991, p. 1290.

Sola, P., Merelli, E., Marasca, R., Poggi, M., and others. Human herpesvirus 6 and multiple sclerosis: survey of anti-HHV-6 antibodies by immunofluorescence analysis and of viral sequences by polymerase chain reaction. *Journal of Neurology, Neurosurgery and Psychiatry* 56(8), 1993, p. 917.

Soldan, S.S., Berti, R., Salem, N, Secchiero, P., Flamand, L., Calabresi, P.A., Brennan, M.B., Maloni, H.W., McFarland, H.F., Lin, H.C., Patnaik, M., Jacobson, S. Association of human herpes virus 6 (HHV-6) with multiple sclerosis: increased IgM response to HHV-6 early antigen and detection of serum HHV-6 DNA, *Nature Medicine*, 3(12), 1997, p. 1394.

Steeper, T.A., Horwitz, C.A., Ablashi, D.V., and others. The spectrum of clinical and laboratory findings resulting from human herpesvirus 6 (HHV-6) in patients with mononucleosis-like illnesses not resulting from Epstein-Barr virus or cytomegalovirus. *American Journal of Clinical Pathology* 93, 1990, p. 776.

Stettner-Gloning, R., Jager, G., Gloning, H., Pontz, B.F., Emmrich, P. Lymphadenopathy in connection with human herpes virus type 6 (HHV-6) infection. *Clinical and Investigative Medicine* 70(1), 1992, p. 59.

Stevens, R.W., Baltch, A.L., and others. Antibody to human endogenous retrovirus peptide in urine of human immunodeficiency virus type 1-positive patients. *Clinical Diagnostic and Laboratory Immunology*, 6(6), 1999, p. 783.

Suga, S., Yoshikawa, T., Asano, Y., Kozawa, T., and others. Clinical and virological analyses of 21 infants with exanthem subitum (roseola infantum) and central nervous system complications. *Annals of Neurology* 33(6), 1993, p. 597.

Sutherland, S., Christofinis, G., O'Grady, J., Williams, R. A serological investigation of human herpesvirus 6 infections in liver transplant recipients and the detection of cross-reacting antibodies to cytomegalovirus. *Journal of Medical Virology* 33, 1991, p. 172.

Tajiri, H., and others. Human herpesvirus 6 infection with liver injury in neonatal hepatitis. *The Lancet*, 335, 1990, p. 863

Tang, Y.W., Espy, M.J., Persing, D.H., Smith, T.F. Molecular evidence and clinical significance of herpesvirus coinfection in the central nervous system. *Journal of Clinical Microbiology* 35(11), 1997, p. 2869.

Tedder, R.S., and others. A novel lymphotropic herpesvirus. *The Lancet* ii, 1987, p. 390.

Thompson, J., Choudhury, S., Kashanchi, F., Doniger, J., and others. A transforming fragment within the direct repeat region of human herpesvirus type 6 that transactivates HIV-1. *Oncogene* 9(4), 1994, p. 1167.

Thomson, B.J., Efstathiou, S., Honess, R.W. Acquisition of the human adeno-associated virus type-2 rep gene by human herpesvirus type-6. *Nature* 351, 1991, p. 78.

Thomson, B.J., Honess, R.W. The right end of the unique region of the genome of human herpesvirus 6 U1102 contains a candidate for immediate early gene enhancer and a homologue of the human cytomegalovirus US22 gene family. *Journal of General Virology* 73(7), 1992, p. 1649.

Torelli, G., and others. Targeted integration of human herpesvirus 6 in the p arm of chromosome 17 of human peripheral mononuclear cells in vivo. *Journal of Medical Virology* 46, 1995, p. 178.

Urnovitz, H.B., and others. HIV-1 antibody serum negativity with urine positivity. *The Lancet* 342, 1993, p. 1458.

Urnovitz, H.B., and others. Urine antibody tests: new insights into the dynamics of HIV-1 infection. *Clinical Chemistry* 45 (9), 1999, p. 1602.

Urnovitz, H.B., Murphy, W.H. Human endogenous retroviruses: nature, occurrence, and clinical implications in human disease. *Clinical Microbiology Reviews* 9 (1), 1996, p. 72.

Urnovitz, H.B., Tuite, J.J., Higashida, J.M., Murphy, W.H. RNAs in the srra of Persian Gulf war veterans have segments homologous to chromosome 22q11.2, *Clinical Diagnostic and Laboratory Immunology* 6 (3), 1999, p. 330.

Valle, B.M., Madueño, J.A., Jurado, R., Fernández-Arcás, N., Muñoz, E. Human herpesvirus-6 and the course of human immunodeficiency virus infection. *Journal of AIDS and Human Retroviruses* 9, 1995, p. 389.

Wade, A.W., McDonald, A.T., Acott, P.D., Lee, S., Crocker, J.F. Human herpes virus-6 or Epstein-Barr virus infection and acute allograft rejection in pediatric kidney transplant recipients: greater risk for immunologically naive recipients. *Transplantation Proceedings*, 30(5), 1998, p. 2091.

Ward, K.N., Gray, J.J. Primary human herpesvirus-6 infection is frequently overlooked as a cause of febrile fits in young children. *Journal of Medical Virology* 42(2), 1994, p. 119.

Ward, K.N., Sheldon, M.J., Gray, J.J. Primary and recurrent cytomegalovirus infections have different effects on human herpesvirus-6 antibodies in immunosuppressed organ graft recipients: absence of virus cross-reactivity and evidence for virus interaction. *Journal of Medical Virology* 34, 1991, p. 258.

Webb, D.W., Bjornson, B.H., Sargent, M.A., Hukin, J., Thomas, E.E. Basal ganglia infarction associated with HHV-6 infection. *Archives of Disease in Childhood*, 76(4), 1997, p. 362.

Wei, X., and others. Viral dynamics in human immunodeficiency virus type 1 infection. *Nature* 373, 1995, p. 117.

Wilborn, F., Brinkmann, V., Schmidt, C.A., Neipel, F., and others. Herpesvirus type 6 in patients undergoing bone marrow transplantation: serologic features and detection by polymerase chain reaction. *Blood* 83(10), 1994, p. 3052.

Wilborn, F., Schmidt, C.A., Brinkmann, V., Jendroska, K., and others. A potential role for human herpesvirus type 6 in nervous system disease. *Journal of Neuroimmunology* 49(1-2), 1994, p. 213.

Yakushijin, Y., Yasukawa, M., Kobayashi, Y. T-cell immune response to human herpesvirus-6 in healthy adults. *Microbiology and Immunology* 35(8), 1991, p. 655.

Yalcin, S., Kuratane, H., Yamaguchi, K., and others. Prevalence of human herpesvirus 6 variant A and B in patients with chronic fatigue syndrome. *Microbiology and Immunology* 38, 1994, p. 587.

Yalcin, S., Mukai, T., Kondo, K., Ami, Y., and others. Experimental infection of cynomolgus and African green monkeys with human herpesvirus 6. *Journal of General Virology* 73 (7), 1992, p. 1673.

Yamanishi, K., and others. Identification of human herpesvirus 6 as a causal agent for exanthem subitum. *The Lancet* i, 1988, p. 1065.

Yolken, R., Torrey, E.F. Viruses, schizophrenia and bipolar disorder. *Clinical Microbiology Reviews* 8 (1), 1995, p. 131.

Yoshikawa, T., and others. Five cases of thrombocytopenia induced by primary human herpesvirus 6 infection. *Acta Paediatrica Japonica* 40(3), 1998, p. 278.

Yoshikawa, T., Kojima, S., Asano, Y. Human herpesvirus-6 infection and bone marrow transplantation. *Leukemia and Lymphoma* 8(1-2), 1992, p. 65.

Yoshikawa, T., Suga, S., Asano, Y., Nakashima, T., and others. A prospective study of human herpesvirus-6 infection in renal transplantation. *Transplantation* 54(5), 1992, p. 879.

Zhou, Y., Chang, C.K., Qian, G., Chandran, B., Wood, C. Trans-activation of the HIV promoter by a cDNA and its genomic clones of human herpesvirus-6. *Virology* 199(2), 1994, p. 311.

Index